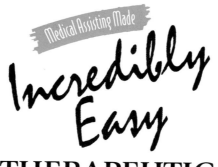

Medical Assisting Made

Incredibly Easy

THERAPEUTIC
COMMUNICATIONS

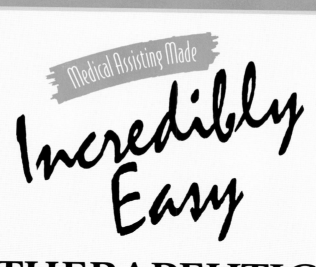

Medical Assisting Made

Incredibly Easy

THERAPEUTIC
COMMUNICATIONS

Kathleen Schreiner, RN, MSHSA

Montgomery County Community College
Pottstown, Pennsylvania

Wolters Kluwer | Lippincott Williams & Wilkins
Health

Philadelphia · Baltimore · New York · London
Buenos Aires · Hong Kong · Sydney · Tokyo

Executive Editor: John Goucher
Managing Editor: Renee Thomas
Senior Marketing Manager: Zhan Caplan
Production Editor: John Larkin
Illustrator: Bot Roda
Designer: Joan Wendt
Compositor: Circle Graphics

First Edition

Library of Congress Cataloging-in-Publication Data

Schreiner, Kathleen.
Therapeutic communications / Kathleen Schreiner.—1st ed.
   p. ; cm.—(Medical assisting made incredibly easy)
ISBN 978-0-7817-7552-6
  1. Communication in medicine. 2. Medical personnel and patient. 3. Medical assistants. I.
Title. II. Series.
  [DNLM: 1. Professional-Patient Relations. 2. Allied Health Personnel. 3. Communication.
W21.5 S378t 2009]
  R118.S34 2009
  610.69'6—dc22

                                        2008016407

Disclaimer

Care has been taken to confirm the accuracy of the information present and to describe generally accepted practices. However, the authors, editors, and publisher are not responsible for errors or omissions or for any consequences from application of the information in this book and make no warranty, expressed or implied, with respect to the currency, completeness, or accuracy of the contents of the publication. Application of this information in a particular situation remains the professional responsibility of the practitioner; the clinical treatments described and recommended may not be considered absolute and universal recommendations.

The authors, editors, and publisher have exerted every effort to ensure that drug selection and dosage set forth in this text are in accordance with the current recommendations and practice at the time of publication. However, in view of ongoing research, changes in government regulations, and the constant flow of information relating to drug therapy and drug reactions, the reader is urged to check the package insert for each drug for any change in indications and dosage and for added warnings and precautions. This is particularly important when the recommended agent is a new or infrequently employed drug.

Some drugs and medical devices presented in this publication have Food and Drug Administration (FDA) clearance for limited use in restricted research settings. It is the responsibility of the health care provider to ascertain the FDA status of each drug or device planned for use in their clinical practice.

To purchase additional copies of this book, call our customer service department at **(800) 638-3030** or fax orders to **(301) 223-2320**. International customers should call **(301) 223-2300**.

Visit Lippincott Williams & Wilkins on the Internet: http://www.lww.com. Lippincott Williams & Wilkins customer service representatives are available from 8:30 am to 6:00 pm, EST.

PREFACE

Medical Assisting Made Incredibly Easy is an exciting new series designed to make learning enjoyable for medical assisting students. Each book in the series uses a light-hearted, humorous approach to presenting information. Maria, a Certified Medical Assistant, guides students through the books, offering helpful tips and insight along the way.

Medical Assisting Made Incredibly Easy takes a practical approach, providing students with the critical information that they need to know, including complete coverage of the core skills they must master in their studies. The series covers all competencies based on the standards and guidelines established for medical assisting by the Commission on Accreditation of Allied Health Educational Programs (CAAHEP) and the Accrediting Bureau of Health Education Schools (ABHES).

About This Book

Medical Assisting Made Incredibly Easy: Therapeutic Communications provides instruction in CAAHEP's Professional Communications competencies and ABHES's Communication competencies (among others). These are among the skills that students must master to pass the test required to become either a Certified Medical Assistant or a Registered Medical Assistant.

Special Features

Medical Assisting Made Incredibly Easy: Therapeutic Communications is designed to be enjoyable to read, as well as highly informative. Each chapter in this book includes special features designed to guide students in their study. These elements will help students identify the most important information in the chapter and to understand all of it.

- *Chapter Checklist* includes a list of skills and other important information that students will gain after reading the material.

- *Chapter Competencies* highlights the ABHES and CAAHEP competencies covered in each chapter.

- *Listen to This* highlights key information pertaining to therapeutic communication.

- *Say It Isn't So* presents realistic, challenging situations with questions that require critical thinking and reinforce key chapter content.

- *Send and Receive* provides examples of dialogue (effective and ineffective) to illustrate key points about communication.

- *Your Turn to Teach* presents tips and highlights opportunities for medical assistants to educate patients.

- *Translating Legal Issues* highlights important legal issues.

- *Translating Ethical Issues* highlights important ethical information.

- *The Voice of Experience* offers advice on how to handle difficult situations you may face in the workplace.

- *Chapter Highlights* summarizes a chapter's key content.

- *Active Learning* provides suggested activities (both individual and small group) for further exploration.

In addition to the above features, this book also includes bolded key terms throughout each chapter and a Glossary in the back of the book, as well as many other boxed features and tables.

Additional Resources

In addition to the text, the following resources are available for students and instructors:

- An **Instructor's Resource CD-ROM** with test generator, PowerPoint slides, and customizable competency evaluation forms helps instructors optimize their teaching. The Instructor's Resource CD-ROM also includes information on where in the book each ABHES and CAAHEP competency is covered.

- A complete set of **Lesson Plans** is also available to instructors.

Medical Assisting Made Incredibly Easy: Therapeutic Communications is designed to make the study of medical assisting fun and effective. The purpose of this book, and the entire *Medical Assisting Made Incredibly Easy* series, is student success!

USER'S GUIDE

Hello, my name is Maria. I'm a Certified Medical Assistant and educator, as well as your guide through this textbook. There are a number of features in this **Medical Assisting Made Incredibly Easy** text to help you learn everything you need to become a successful medical assistant. Read through this User's Guide to orient yourself to everything the text has to offer. Good luck in your medical assisting studies!

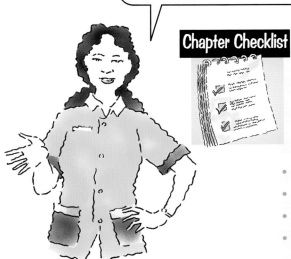

Chapter Checklist

- Demonstrate an understanding of human growth and development
- Explain cognitive development theory
- List and describe Freud's three major systems or forces
- Define the reality principle and the pleasure principle
- List and describe Erikson's eight psychosocial crises
- Explain the principle of mutuality
- Define operant conditioning
- Discuss the impact of reinforcement on behavior
- Explain the significance of understanding developmental theories as they relate to approaches to communication
- Demonstrate a basic understanding of the challenges of communicating with each age group
- Describe a holistic approach to health care communication
- List communication techniques for working with children
- Describe communication techniques for working with adolescents
- Identify communication techniques for working with adults
- List and describe the therapeutic communication techniques for an older population

Chapter Checklists orient you to the material that's covered in the current chapter.

Chapter Competencies

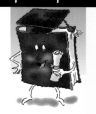

- Recognize and respond to verbal and nonverbal communication (CAAHEP Competency 3.c.1.b. and 3.c.1.c.; ABHES Competency 2.i. and 2.l.)
- Interview effectively (ABHES Competency 2.f.)
- Be a "team player" (ABHES Competency 1.c.)
- Be courteous and diplomatic (ABHES Competency 1.h.)
- Be attentive, listen, and learn (ABHES Competency 2.a.)
- Be impartial and show empathy when dealing with patients (ABHES Competency 2.b.)
- Demonstrate fundamental writing skills (ABHES Competency 2.o.)

Chapter Competencies tell you which skills are covered in each chapter, as outlined by CAAHEP and ABHES.

Listen to This boxes highlight key information pertaining to therapeutic communication.

Listen to This

CULTURAL COMPETENCE CHECKLIST

When interacting with patients of different cultures, keep this cultural competence checklist in mind. Review each of the factors listed below to see how culturally competent your patient interactions are.

Am I being sensitive to the patient's:

- beliefs, values, traditions, and practices
- culturally defined health-related needs
- culturally based beliefs
- culturally based attitudes

Say it Isn't So

WRITING PERSONAL NOTES TO PATIENTS

What if a patient also happens to be a friend? Would it be acceptable to include a personal note on any professional communication sent from the medical office?

You may have friends, family members, or acquaintances who come to your office to see the physician. Because they are patients, it's also probable that there will be situations in which you need to send a letter, note, or other written communication to them. You should not write differently to patients who are friends. As a medical assistant, you should write just as professionally to all patients, whether you know them personally or not.

Say It Isn't So boxes present realistic, challenging situations and give you a chance to apply your critical thinking skills.

Send and Receive

BREAKING DOWN COMMUNICATION BARRIERS

Send and Receive boxes give you examples of effective and ineffective dialogue.

Imagine that you're a medical assistant interviewing a patient who speaks very little English. What would you do? How would you communicate? Here are some examples of ineffective and effective dialogue.

Ineffective:

- "What brings you here today, Ms. Garcia?" Ms. Garcia looks puzzled. Speaking louder, the medical assistant repeats, "I said what brings you here today, Ms. Garcia?"
- "According to your chart, it looks like the physician [ ] a herniated intervertebral [ ] encing unremitting pain or [ ] es?"
- [ ] non–English-speaking [ ] ak in simple sentences. When

Your Turn to Teach

ACTIVELY LISTEN

A patient sits in the examination room with his head down, arms folded, and shoulders slouched. You must collect some basic information about the patient before the physician sees him. Practice your active listening skills by following these steps:

- The patient's body language clearly says that he is uncomfortable and not feeling well. To help the patient feel as comfortable as possible, make sure the room is private and quiet.
- Address the patient by his name. Make eye contact. Be warm, courteous, and respectful. Face the patient using an open stance. Ask questions clearly.
- Give the patient your full attention when talking *and* listening. Allow the patient to speak without interrupting.
- Be aware of how the patient communicates nonverbally. What [ ] gestur[ ] have? [ ]
- Ackno[ ] listen! Do no[ ]

Your Turn to Teach boxes provide helpful information about patient education.

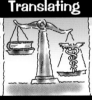

Translating

Legal Issues

E-MAIL CONFIDENTIALITY

E-mail is a quick and convenient way to communicate with others in your office. But there is one important fact to keep in mind when using e-mail. The messages you send and receive can't be guaranteed to be private and confidential. To help keep your e-mail messages as confidential and private as possible, follow these tips:

- Send only work-related e-mail messages. Do not send personal messages using your work e-mail address.
- Read about your e-mail program's encryption feature and activate it. Encryption is a process that scrambles messages so that they can't be read until they reach the recipient.
- Use the out-of-office-assistant feature to alert senders when you're out of the office or on vacation. This lets senders know that you'll not be reading their messages immediately.

Translating Legal Issues boxes highlight important legal issues.

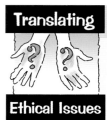

IMPAIRED COWORKERS

The National Association of Social Workers website states, "An estimated 20 percent of workers suffer from some type of impairment, which may include substance abuse, psychological stresses due to aging, physical illness, financial hardship, extreme working conditions, marital and family difficulties, or chronic psychological disorders." These impairments may create ethical situations for health care practitioners.

For example, suppose you're the office manager for a well respected family physician in a small town. He is 70 years old and is starting to show signs of senility. He is forgetful and has even been disoriented and confused a few times. No one seems to have noticed. You respect the physician, but you're concerned that his condition may be placing patients' health and safety at risk. How should you handle this ethical dilemma?

Any time a physician or coworker's impairment has the potential to affect the quality of care being provided to patients, it's your ethical responsibility to report your concerns to the appropriate authority. In this particular situation, you should report the physician's condition to the administration of the hospital where he has privileges or to the state board of medicine. The physician's family may be involved in the situation as well.

Translating Ethical Issues boxes highlight important ethical information.

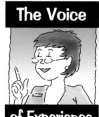

GUIDING PRINCIPLES OF THERAPEUTIC COMMUNICATION

Q: *What does it mean to remain professional in all relationships with patients? How do I know what is professional and what is not?*

A: Remaining professional means never forgetting that you have a responsibility to the patient, the physician, and your employer. Even if the patient wants to discuss topics that do not relate to his care, such as rumor or gossip, your responsibility is to be polite, but professional, and always try to guide the conversation back to the topic of your patient's health.

The Voice of Experience boxes provide advice on how to handle difficult situations you may face in the workplace.

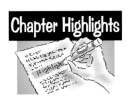

Chapter Highlights

- The components of the patient interview include obtaining a medical history, assessing signs and symptoms, gathering details about the chief complaint and present illness, and documenting the patient's history.
- Verbal communication is sending and receiving messages using words or language.
- Nonverbal communication, also known as body language, involves exchanging messages without using words. Forms of nonverbal communication include body position, facial expressions, touch, and gestures.
- Active listening is an important part of communication. You can listen actively by being engaged with what the other person is saying, supplying your full attention, and paying attention to nonverbal clues.
- When conducting patient interviews, it's helpful to use a mixture of open-ended and closed-ended questions, as well as indirect statements.
- When obtaining and recording a patient history, remember to maintain eye contact, use language the patient can understand, and listen actively to the patient's responses.
- Know the difference between sympathy and empathy. Sympathy is feeling sorry for someone, but empathy is the ability to [understand anot]her person's feelings. It's impor[tant to use more t]han sympathy for patients.

Chapter Highlights summarizes a chapter's key content.

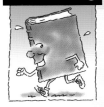

Active Learning

COMMUNICATING WITHOUT WORDS

Imagine that you're asked to escort a patient back to the examination room. The physician has also asked you to identify the reason for the patient's visit (chief complaint). However, suppose the patient does not speak any English. How would you communicate with him?

With a partner, act out the roles of non–English-speaking patient and medical assistant. Without using words, escort the patient to an "examination room" and obtain the patient's chief complaint. Then, switch roles and repeat.

Finally, share with the rest of the class the various methods you and your partner used to communicate.

Active Learning provides suggested activities for further exploration.

CULTURAL DIFFERENCES IN DIET

Using the information presented in *Cultural Differences in Nutrition* on page 141 as a starting point, choose a culture that you know very little about and research cultural differences in diet. Create a list with two columns to identify areas in which your own culture's diet is similar to and different from the diet of the cultural group you've chosen to research.

REVIEWERS

Nina Beaman
Bryant and Stratton College
Richmond, Virginia

Deeann Knox
Ball State University and St Francis College of Health Professions
Fort Wayne, Indiana

Helen Houser
Phoenix College
Phoenix, Arizona

Maureen Messier
Bradford Hall Career Institute
Southington, Connecticut

Amy Semenchuk
Rockford Business College
Rockford, Illinois

Lynn Slack
Kaplan Career Institute
Pittsburgh, Pennsylvania

Nina Thierer
Ivy Tech Community College
Fort Wayne, Indiana

TABLE OF CONTENTS

PREFACE   v

USER'S GUIDE   ix

REVIEWERS   xv

Chapter 1
DEVELOPING SELF-AWARENESS   1

Chapter 2
THE COMMUNICATION CYCLE   26

Chapter 3
COMMUNICATION ACROSS THE LIFESPAN   53

Chapter 4
BUILDING BRIDGES: COMMUNICATING
WITH PATIENTS   95

Chapter 5
THE CULTURALLY DIVERSE WORKPLACE   131

Chapter 6
TECHNIQUES TO TACKLE COMMUNICATION
CHALLENGES   165

Chapter 7
PROVIDING PATIENT WELLNESS
AND EDUCATION   207

Chapter 8
WRITTEN COMMUNICATIONS AND
TECHNOLOGY   240

Chapter 9
USING PROFESSIONAL COMMUNICATION SKILLS IN
THE WORKPLACE   271

GLOSSARY   301

INDEX   311

EXPANDED TABLE OF CONTENTS

PREFACE   v

USER'S GUIDE   ix

REVIEWERS   xv

Chapter 1
DEVELOPING SELF-AWARENESS   1
  Self-Concept: Who Are You, Really?   2
  Know Thyself!   6
  The Role of Self-Concept   8
  Strengths and Weaknesses   12
  Reactions and Responses   14
  Building Atmospheres that Foster Self-Esteem   16
  Maslow's Hierarchy of Needs   19
  Developing Skills for Professional and Personal Growth   22
  Developing Insight   23

Chapter 2
THE COMMUNICATION CYCLE   26
  Communication: It's More than Just Talking   27
  The Communication Cycle   30
  Context: The What, Where, When, and How of
  Communication   33
  To Speak or Not to Speak—Verbal and Nonverbal
  Communication   34
  Listening   42
  Putting Your Communication Skills to Work   44
  Developing Your Communication Skills   48

Chapter 3

COMMUNICATION ACROSS THE LIFESPAN   53
  Growth, Development, and Behavior and Its Impact
  on Communication   54
  Piaget   55
  Sigmund Freud   56
  Erik Erikson   60
  B. F. Skinner   67
  Different Age Groups Communicate Differently   69
  Chatting with Children   73
  Talking with Teens   76
  Communicating with Adults   81
  Communicating with Older Adults   84

Chapter 4

BUILDING BRIDGES: COMMUNICATING
WITH PATIENTS   95
  Patient Interviews   96
  Challenges to Communication   106
  Defense Mechanisms   112
  Problem-Solving Skills   114
  Legal and Ethical Issues   116
  Confidentiality   121
  Releasing Information and Initiating or Terminating
  Treatment   121

Chapter 5

THE CULTURALLY DIVERSE WORKPLACE   131
  Heredity, Culture, and Environment   132
  Communicating with a Culturally Diverse Population   137
  The Cultural Guidebook   138
  Are You Culturally Competent?   152
  Providing Culturally Competent Care   156

Chapter 6

TECHNIQUES TO TACKLE COMMUNICATION
CHALLENGES   165
  Communication Challenges   166
  Drug and Alcohol Addiction   167
  Grief and Loss Reactions   171
  HIV/AIDS   179
  Stress and Anxiety   183
  Anger and Aggression   185
  Disabilities   190
  Depression and Suicidal Feelings   194
  Abuse and Harassment   199

Chapter 7

PROVIDING PATIENT WELLNESS
AND EDUCATION   207
  Promoting Health Maintenance and Disease
  Prevention   208
  Stress   212
  Nutrition   218
  Exercise   223
  Medications   226
  Understanding Office Procedures   230
  Community Resources   236

Chapter 8

WRITTEN COMMUNICATIONS
AND TECHNOLOGY   240
  Written Communication Is Important   241
  How Computer Technology Helps   258
  Communication Equipment   264
  Patient Brochures   267

Chapter 9

USING PROFESSIONAL COMMUNICATION SKILLS
IN THE WORKPLACE   271
  Communicating with Your Health Care Team   272
  Workplace Dynamics and Office Procedures   274
  Managing Workplace Conflict   280
  Supervisory Styles   290
  Employment Communication Skills   292
  Communication and Professional Growth   297

GLOSSARY   301

INDEX   311

Chapter 1

DEVELOPING SELF-AWARENESS

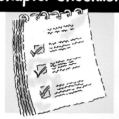

Chapter Checklist

- Define self-concept

- Describe the role self-concept plays in determining who we are and what we think, what we do, and what we can become

- Explain the significance of assessing our strengths and weaknesses in relationship to our self-concept

- Determine how the responses that we receive from others as a result of our behavior influence our self-concept

- Develop an understanding of the importance of verbal and nonverbal messages

- Define feedback

- Describe atmospheres that build self-esteem

- Exhibit a multidimensional approach to building the physical, mental, psychological, and social characteristics that are consistent with a positive self-image

- List Maslow's hierarchy of needs

- Develop interpersonal skills and use therapeutic communication techniques

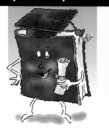

Chapter Competencies

- Be attentive; listen and learn (ABHES Competency 2.a.)

- Recognize and respond to verbal communications (CAAHEP Competency 3.c.1.b.)

- Recognize and respond to verbal and nonverbal communication (ABHES Competency 2.i.)

- Principles of verbal and nonverbal communication (ABHES Competency 2.k.)

- Recognition and response to verbal and nonverbal communication (ABHES Competency 2.1.)
- Recognize and respond to nonverbal communications (CAAHEP Competency 3.c.1.c.)
- Be impartial and show empathy when dealing with patients (ABHES Competency 2.b.)
- Project a positive attitude (ABHES Competency 1.a.)
- Evidence a responsible attitude (ABHES Competency 1.g.)

You're probably wondering why a book about therapeutic communication would begin with a chapter about self-awareness. The messages that we communicate are affected in large part by how we feel about ourselves, our surroundings, and those around us. To communicate effectively as a medical assistant, you must be able to understand yourself first. When you know yourself, you'll be able to connect with others more easily! By being aware of your behavior and actions, you'll be in a position to have a positive influence on those you come in contact with.

In this chapter, you'll learn about self-concept and the different types of self. You'll also learn how self-concept and self-esteem influence each other. You'll see that a positive self-concept and high self-esteem are valuable tools to have when interacting with others.

Self-Concept: Who Are You, Really?

Your self-concept includes all the feelings, beliefs, and values you associate with yourself. Why is this important? When your self-concept is positive, you're more likely to act in ways that other people will see as positive. You might smile more, or hold the door open for a stranger. Your feelings of personal worth affect how you convey your worth to others. It also affects the way others react to you. An understanding of self-concept is a helpful tool to have as a health care professional. It will help you communicate with and relate to patients more effectively.

ONE SELF-CONCEPT IS MADE OF MANY PARTS

Simply put, your **self-concept** is the mental image or picture you have of yourself. Some psychologists think that your self-concept is the single most influential factor that determines your behavior. Depending on how positive or negative it is, your self-concept can either strengthen or weaken your personal growth throughout life.

Your self-concept can be broken down into these specific components:

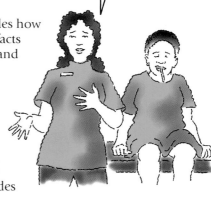

When your self-concept is healthy and strong, it makes it easier to help others.

- *Personal identity.* This component includes how you describe yourself in terms of basic facts (e.g., your age or cultural background) and traits (e.g., kind, intelligent, driven).

- *Body image.* This component includes how you see yourself physically (e.g., the color of your hair and eyes, your height and weight).

- *Self-esteem.* This component includes the level of respect you have for yourself.

- *Role performance.* This component includes how well you fulfill the different roles you play in life.

When you nurture and maintain a positive self-concept, your personal identity is positive, your body image is positive, your self-esteem is high, and your role performance is effective.

IDENTIFY YOURSELF!

Your self-concept is determined, in part, by your sense of identity. Your sense of identity is the way you identify yourself. It's your sense of your capabilities and limitations. Every decision you make depends on whether you see yourself succeeding or failing.

There are some key questions that reveal your sense of identity. Ask yourself the following questions:

- How would I describe myself to others?
- What are some of my personal characteristics and traits?
- What are my strengths?
- What are my fears?
- What roles do I have?
- Am I satisfied with my roles and how I fulfill them?
- Who or what has influenced the expectations I have for myself?

Being aware of your sense of identity is a good first step in becoming self-aware. You might find out that you have strengths you never noticed before. You might also find out that you're not as good at some things as you once thought you were. Whether your sense of identity is positive or negative, just knowing you have one can help you to think about and possibly even change it.

WHERE DOES YOUR SELF-CONCEPT COME FROM?

Your self-concept does not suddenly appear during adolescence or adulthood. Your self-concept begins to form at an early age. It's usually well established by the time you're 6-years-old. Because self-concept generally takes shape while you're young, early interactions with certain "significant" people in your life are critically important to developing a healthy self-concept. Here's a summary of how your self-concept forms.

1. As an infant, your first positive feelings form. This occurs as your caregivers meet your basic needs and as you experience warmth and affection.

2. As a growing child, you absorb other peoples' attitudes regarding your behavior. If a close family member praised drawings you made as a young child, you might begin to think of yourself as a creative person. The cues you get from close family and friends lay the foundation for self-concept. As you continue to grow, your behavior reflects those early beliefs about yourself.

3. As you mature, you become more and more aware of the standards of society. Even if you did not put a napkin on your lap before you sat down to dinner with your family, you might pick up this habit after seeing others do it in a restaurant. After picking up the habit, you might begin to view yourself as someone with good table manners. Being aware of the world around you influences your self-concept throughout your lifetime.

What affects the formation of self-concept? Remember that self-concept is learned, so it can be influenced, reinforced, modified, or even completely changed by many things. For example, here's a list of several factors that help create a positive self-concept in childhood:

- emotional warmth and acceptance
- effective structure and discipline
- clearly defined standards and limits
- adequately defined roles for both older and younger family members
- established expectations

- rewards for acceptable behavior and consequences for unacceptable behavior
- encouragement of competence and self-confidence
- help in meeting challenges
- appropriate role models
- a stimulating and responsive environment

Contemporary theories agree that you form your self-concept largely by comparing yourself to people who matter to you. But it's also formed by looking at yourself as you believe other people see you.

INFLUENCE OF SELF-CONCEPT

Once it's established, your self-concept acts as a kind of filter. Everything you see, hear, evaluate, and understand goes through this filter. Input from peers, family members, friends, and role models affects your self-concept. The nature of your self-concept defines the effects of this input.

For example, imagine that a coworker has just made a comment about the way you interacted with a patient. Your coworker tells you that Mr. Blackman is hard of hearing and that you should have written down more of the physician's instructions for him in case he couldn't hear you. If your self-concept is generally positive and healthy, you might interpret the remark as a helpful pointer that will make your next interaction with a patient even better. But if your self-concept is weak, you might be very hurt by the remark, or you might decide that the coworker was trying to hurt you.

We like to put those kinds of charts in this file over here.

Thanks for letting me know. I'll do that from now on.

If your self-concept is positive, you can turn comments from coworkers and employers into opportunities to improve your work!

In fact, the coworker could have either been trying to be helpful or hurtful. The other person's reasons for making a remark actually matter very little in comparison to how you interpret what is said. Having a healthy self-concept allows you to stay in control of your feelings. Your self-concept can help you to filter out the negative and retain the positive.

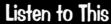

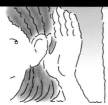

WHY IS SELF-CONCEPT IMPORTANT?

Here's a list summarizing why self-concept is important.
- It affects how you feel about yourself.
- It affects how you feel about others.
- It affects how others feel about you.
- It affects how you interact with others.
- It affects your behavior from an early age.
- It's a reflection of your sense of identity.

Know Thyself!

Your self-concept is determined by your own definition of self. Think about that! How would you define *you?* There are many, many sides to you. You behave and react differently in different situations. You have various likes and dislikes. In other words, *you* have many components of self. And these components are tied closely to your self-concept.

COMPONENTS OF SELF

The components of self, or the different sides of *you,* include your:
- *Material self.* This component includes your physical body and your possessions.
- *Psychological self.* When you analyze your thoughts and ideas, you're experiencing your psychological self.
- *Emotional self.* Your emotional self refers to the way you feel personally about your experiences.
- *Social self.* The way you interact with others makes up your social self.
- *Ideal self.* This component refers to the person you think you should be or who you would like to be someday.
- *Public self.* This component represents how you want others to see you. You may have many public selves, depending on the circle of people with whom you have contact. Your public self is the image you want others to have about you, or your reputation.

- *Real self.* This is your inner, natural self. It's authentic and spontaneous. Put simply, your "real self" is who you are when no one is watching.

DEVELOPING SELF-ACCEPTANCE

Also related closely to self-concept is your feeling of self-acceptance. Do you accept who you are? Do you accept your strengths and limitations? Before your self-esteem can be high, you must be willing to accept yourself as you are—not as who you think you should be, or who you plan to be in 6 months. To truly accept yourself, you need to strike a balance between your real self, ideal self, and public self. All three must not only be balanced—you also have to feel good about each of these components!

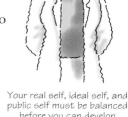

LAYING THE FOUNDATION FOR SELF-ESTEEM

With positive self-acceptance comes high self-esteem. But what, exactly, creates high self-esteem? Two factors that can help you lay the foundation for high self-esteem include:

- success in encounters and experiences
- acceptance from parents and significant people

Your real self, ideal self, and public self must be balanced before you can develop self-acceptance.

Success and Competency

Building self-esteem is like constructing a tower. Your first successes lay the basic foundation. Each additional success makes the tower higher and higher. However, early failures in your life can prevent you from laying a strong foundation. Repeated failures make it more and more difficult to build high self-esteem.

An important step in building high self-esteem is to recognize your successes—even small ones—as they occur. When you're a young child, your "significant" people like your parents, guardians, or close relatives, do this for you. But as you grow and mature, you learn and develop skills that allow you to be aware of your successes. As your life progresses, each success builds on itself. You become more and more capable as your self-esteem grows higher and higher.

Parental Acceptance

High self-esteem is also connected to parental acceptance. Parental acceptance is part of the supportive environment needed when you're developing and growing. As you mature, unresolved conflicts between you and your parents can affect your self-esteem and, thus, your self-concept, in a negative way.

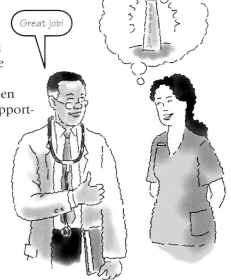

For example, strong parental support for a favorite hobby or activity helps you feel good about yourself and what you're doing. Being able to start new activities, go to new places, or learn new things often depends on whether your parents are support-ive or not.

You can also receive "parental accep-tance" from people other than your par-ents. Teachers, group leaders, mentors, and other role models are important sources of acceptance. The responses you get from them have a big impact on your self-concept.

The Role of Self-Concept

As you have seen, self-concept plays a strong role in determin-ing who you are and what you think, what you do, and who you can become. You've also learned that to have a strong self-concept, you must also have high self-esteem.

GOOD CONDITIONS MAKE SELF-ESTEEM GROW

In the last section, you learned about the kinds of things that lay the foundation for self-esteem. In 1981, Harris Clemes and Reynold Bean outlined four conditions that are necessary for self-esteem to grow:

- connection to others
- appreciation of uniqueness
- empowerment
- model behavior

Connection to Others

Being able to connect to others in a positive way is an impor-tant part of building self-esteem. Making this kind of positive connection is valuable for two reasons. First, it's satisfying to you. Second, it's satisfying to others. And the satisfaction that others feel as a result of such a connection is communicated back to you.

For example, a patient may walk into the medical office visibly upset or concerned. Being aware of the patient's emotional state, you might immediately approach the patient and ask if they would like some water, tissues, or even a quiet room. Making connections like this with patients shows that you're taking the time to be aware of others and their needs. It also affirms your positive sense of self-esteem and self-concept.

When you connect with others, you must be aware of the ways you express yourself and how you affect the feelings of others. You do this by using both verbal and nonverbal communication skills.

- **Verbal communication skills** are the skills you use when you use words to communicate with others. Being able to communicate effectively using words is a vital part of connecting positively to others.
- **Nonverbal communication skills** are the skills you use when you use body language, facial expressions, or physical gestures to communicate with others.

It's also critical that your verbal and nonverbal communication messages complement each other. For example, you wouldn't say, "Good morning, Mrs. Smith. It's wonderful to see you today!" with a scowl on your face and your arms folded. Instead, you would probably greet her with a bright smile.

When you're secure within yourself, it's much easier to be open and honest in your communication with others. It also makes it easier to use effective verbal and nonverbal communication skills to communicate the right messages.

Appreciation of Uniqueness

Nobody knows *you* better than you. Being aware of and appreciating your own uniqueness plays a strong role in building self-esteem. It means that you're able to acknowledge and respect the things that make you special and different. Appreciating your uniqueness also happens when others recognize your unique qualities.

Just as important, though, is your ability to recognize and accept the uniqueness of others. Acceptance forms a critical part in appreciating uniqueness. Accepting means recognizing a person as another human being with strong needs, feelings, and purposes that need to be acknowledged and understood. Accepting others' uniqueness means being able to listen to and communicate effectively with them. When interacting with others, a medical assistant must show both empathy and respect.

Empathize, Do Not Sympathize

Empathy is the ability to identify with another person's world, experience, or situation. When you empathize with another person, you see the situation from the other person's point of view. Empathy is different from *sympathy* in that when you empathize, you can still step away and offer professional care in your role as a medical assistant. Sympathizing, on the other hand, requires you to become emotionally involved with the patient who is hurting. You may feel sorry for them. When you sympathize, it can be hard to step back and offer care as a professional.

Empathizing helps you better understand what another person is going through without projecting any of your own attitudes or values into the situation. Some might refer to this as being able to "walk in someone else's shoes."

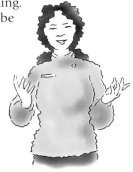

Empathy helps you understand what someone else is going through. As a medical assistant, it's important to have empathy, rather than sympathy, for patients.

Show Some Respect

Respect is the ability to sincerely communicate to another person that you believe in her worth and dignity. You may not be able to like every person you come into contact with as a medical assistant, but part of your job is to show respect to each person you deal with. This can be a tough challenge. It's not easy to treat rude patients or coworkers with respect. In those tough times, it's important to remind yourself that showing respect to others is a way of developing respect for yourself. Communicating with respect allows you to contribute to your own self-worth and boost your self-esteem.

Empowerment

Empowerment happens when you have the resources, opportunity, and capability to positively influence the circumstances of your life as well as the lives of others. Just as the word suggests, *empowerment* is a powerful tool in building self-esteem. There are two ways in which you can use empowerment as a medical assistant:

- influencing others
- empowering others

Influencing Others

When you influence other people in a positive way, you help build your self-esteem. As a medical assistant, you'll often find yourself dealing with patients who test the strength of your self-esteem. In these instances, remember to address the situation rather than the personality of the patient.

For example, you might have a patient in the waiting room who has a short temper. After a short wait in the office, the patient becomes irritable and angry and starts asking in a loud voice when they will be seen. Rather than pointing out that the patient is simply being impatient, allow them to express their concern. Then, calmly explain that the physician makes sure that each patient gets the amount of time necessary to address his or her health care needs. By doing so, you might positively influence the patient to become less impatient. You empower yourself to take control of the situation. If you offer the patient the opportunity to schedule an appointment for another day, you're also empowering the patient to take control of their situation. Offering the patient more control shows that you respect them and that you have respect for yourself.

Empowering Others

As a medical assistant, you have the challenge of sending patients the message that they can make decisions and assume responsibility for the consequences of those decisions. Doing this in an atmosphere of respect empowers patients and enables their self-concept and self-esteem to grow. For example, helping patients to see the importance of eating a balanced diet and exercising regularly helps them take control of their health. And a patient who is empowered to take control of his own health has increased self-esteem.

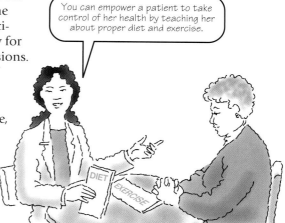

You can empower a patient to take control of her health by teaching her about proper diet and exercise.

Model Behavior

Using behavior models also helps build self-esteem. Positive behavior models are people whose examples help you establish your own:

- meaningful values
- goals
- ideals
- standards

Observing these role models and their actions influences your own behavior.

As a medical assistant, you'll need to seek out positive behavior models so you can learn how to communicate effectively. You should know that it's important to choose role models who use appropriate therapeutic communication techniques. Look to role models who exhibit behavior that is genuine, concrete, and influential.

Genuinely Speaking

When you speak to other people in a sincere, nondefensive, and honest manner, you're more likely to get the same type of responses in return. This goes for your communication with patients as well as for your interactions with coworkers and supervisors. Choose role models who express their honest feelings in a constructive way, without assigning blame or criticizing.

Giving Concrete Answers

Your role models should be professionals who are committed to giving specific, factual information to patients. And just as important, patients need to be able to understand the facts that are being told to them. Different types of patients pose different challenges. Small children, for example, do not generally understand most of the medical terms you may be used to using. You need to be able to give concrete information to children without telling them things that are untrue. Learn from other professionals who tell patients the information they need to know as simply and as directly as possible.

Using Your Influence

If your role models are charismatic and influential, you'll want to pattern your behavior after theirs. By learning how to become influential, you can have a positive effect on patients and coworkers.

For example, by using your high self-esteem and positive self-concept, you can create a sort of magnetic connection between you and a patient. Engage the patient with your dynamic personality! By doing so, the patient will be more inclined to listen to and consider what you have to say.

Likewise, you can also use your influence to communicate more effectively with coworkers. If you have the respect of your coworkers, you'll be able to use your influence to help people discuss their concerns with one another and resolve their differences.

Strengths and Weaknesses

Looking honestly at your strengths and weaknesses may not be easy, but it's a critical skill to have in developing your self-concept.

STRENGTHS

Strengths can be any physical, mental, emotional, or social skills, talents, abilities, or personal characteristics that help you function effectively in your world. In the "world" of the medical office, here are some examples of strengths that are useful to have as a medical assistant:

- *Physical characteristics.* These are the characteristics displayed by your exterior self. As a medical assistant, the physical image you portray influences how patients interact with you. Is your uniform clean and tidy? Is your hair neatly groomed? Do you have good personal hygiene habits?

- *Emotional characteristics.* These are the characteristics displayed by your interior self. Your emotional characteristics might include your ability to be capable, compassionate, friendly, and respectful to others.

- *Social characteristics.* These characteristics include your ability to express yourself with confidence. Your strong social characteristics help you listen attentively to, appreciate, and acknowledge the needs of others.

WEAKNESSES

A weakness is a lack of talent, knowledge, or ability that keeps you from functioning effectively. A weakness in any area may make it difficult to interact with other people. It's important to be aware of any weaknesses you may have. If possible, do what you can to strengthen the weaknesses you identify.

For example, if you lack knowledge about a particular medical condition or treatment, use resources to increase your understanding. You might seek additional information by reviewing a textbook or reading an article in a professional journal. If your weakness is that you lack confidence with certain skills, practice the skills until your confidence improves. In short, find ways to turn your weaknesses into strengths.

Taking the time to read up on a subject is a great way to turn a weakness into a strength!

WHERE DO YOUR STRENGTHS AND WEAKNESSES COME FROM?

But how are your strengths and weaknesses determined? The environment in which you're raised influences how you perceive your strengths and weaknesses.

Many of your emotional and social characteristics depend on the environment in which you grow and develop. Earlier in this chapter, you read about the importance of "significant" people in your life. Your interactions with these "significant" people, including your family members, teachers, peers, and even strangers, play a part in how you see your strengths and weaknesses.

The values of the society in which you live also have an impact on your strengths and weaknesses. For example, different cultures attach different values to certain body types. In some societies, full-figured women are considered beautiful (a strength). However, in other societies, having a full figure may be associated with being overweight (a weakness). It's important to keep in mind that society's values can affect the way you perceive your own strengths and weaknesses. However, that does not mean you have to accept those values!

Reactions and Responses

You send both verbal and nonverbal messages to others when you communicate. People respond and react to those messages, and these responses provide you with feedback. The responses and reactions you receive from other people influence your self-concept in a variety of ways.

SELF-CONCEPT IS A CIRCULAR EFFECT

When you communicate with others—verbally or nonverbally—you send out messages in your words, gestures, expressions, and body language. The person you're communicating with reacts and responds to those messages in many ways. The ways in which others react and respond to your messages affects your self-concept. As a result, your future behavior toward others is affected.

Let's say you walk into your workplace one morning and decide to greet everyone with a cheery "Good morning!" One of your fellow employees smiles back and says, "Good morning to you, too!" Another employee scowls and says, "Please, I'd rather not speak this early in the morning." The following morning, you'll more than likely exchange another cheerful "Good morning!" with the first employee. But you'll probably think twice before saying "Good morning" to the scowling employee again.

Based on their frame of reference, people interpret the feedback they receive from others and use the feedback to formulate or develop their "sense of self." In other words, your self-concept is influenced strongly by the way others respond to your behavior. And the way your self-concept is influenced affects your future behavior toward others.

FEEDBACK HELPS YOU LEARN

The responses and reactions you receive from others are called **feedback**. As you just learned, feedback affects your self-concept and influences your future behavior. It also gives you an opportunity to think about how you communicate with others and what this says about your own self-concept. Remember, the way you communicate with others is connected to how you think of yourself. Feedback is like a mirror for your self-concept.

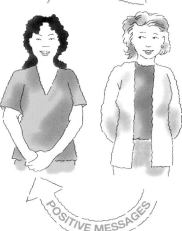

The circular effect of self-concept means that you'll get back what you send out! If you want to receive positive messages, you need to give them to others.

Positive Feedback Is Important!

When somebody responds favorably to something you have said or done, it strengthens your self-concept and self-esteem. Following the circular effect principle, you should try to communicate with others in a way that provides positive feedback for behaviors you want to foster.

The Sender Is Important!

The feedback you receive from significant others has a stronger effect than feedback from strangers. The feedback you receive from a parent is more meaningful than the feedback you might receive from a casual acquaintance. When you receive feedback, think carefully about the sender. If the sender is someone you would not want to emulate, such as a coworker who is rude to patients, you might want to ignore the feedback. But if the feedback comes from a patient you've always admired for his good nature, you might want to use that feedback to improve your own behaviors and self-concept.

Frequency Is Important!

The more you hear or see a reaction, the greater the impact on your behavior. Remember the "Good morning!" example? If you continue to offer your cheerful "Good morning!" to the first employee and she continues to offer it back to you, what will happen? You're both receiving positive feedback, so you and the employee will probably always start the morning with a cheery "Good morning!"

Consistency Is Important!

Consistency has to do with new information falling in line with information and beliefs you have already collected or developed. If the feedback you receive is in line with your own beliefs or perceptions, you're more likely to accept it. However, if some feedback is not consistent with your belief system, that does not make it wrong or useless. Use that feedback to test your own system. See if the feedback can help you improve upon the self-concept you're developing.

Building Atmospheres that Foster Self-Esteem

Many people spend a significant amount of time at work each week. It makes sense, then, that your working environment has a strong effect on your self-concept. Building an atmosphere in the workplace that strengthens self-concept is a critical part of being a successful medical assistant.

MULTIDIMENSIONAL APPROACH

Before you can create a healthy atmosphere at work, you need to start with yourself! Take a multidimensional approach to improving your self-concept. Use the information you've learned in this chapter to build the physical, mental, psychological, and social characteristics that you need to have a positive self-image. Ask yourself:

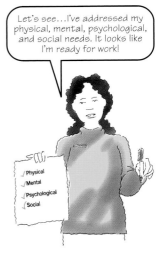

Let's see...I've addressed my physical, mental, psychological, and social needs. It looks like I'm ready for work!

✓ Physical
✓ Mental
✓ Psychological
✓ Social

- Am I getting enough exercise?
- Am I eating a healthy, balanced diet?
- Do I take time for myself?
- Do I have a hobby or favorite activity that I do regularly?
- Do I get together with friends?

By taking care of all parts of *you*, you prepare yourself in the best way possible to work effectively and successfully with others.

GETTING POSITIVE

By using your therapeutic communication skills, you help build a positive atmosphere in your work environment. Here are some guidelines to follow as you begin to build a positive atmosphere:

- Set and enforce clear limits for behavior between yourself and patients. However, allow enough freedom of choice

Send and Receive

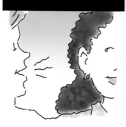

PROVIDING POSITIVE FEEDBACK

Not only do you receive feedback, you also give feedback to others. You may be the first person patients come in contact with upon entering the medical office. As you interact with patients, you'll need to focus on providing positive feedback. Here are some examples of ineffective and effective dialogue between a medical assistant and a patient.

Ineffective:

- As the medical assistant leads the patient back to an examination room, the patient smiles and comments that the weather outside is particularly nice today. The medical assistant, clearly annoyed, responds with: "Well, I wouldn't know, because I've been stuck in the office all day."

- In the examination room, the medical assistant asks the patient about the reason for her office visit. The patient says she's been experiencing headaches and other symptoms for the past five days. The medical assistant asks accusingly, "Why didn't you come in as soon as you started experiencing the symptoms?"

How do you think the medical assistant's feedback would make the patient feel? Would the patient be likely to be open and honest in her other responses to the medical assistant's questions? The circular effect of feedback on self-concept is powerful. And because feedback also influences future behavior, it's especially important for health care professionals to provide positive and encouraging feedback. Patients need to feel that you genuinely care about them and their health concerns.

Effective:

- The medical assistant greets the patient with a smile and leads her back to the examination room. When the patient comments on the nice weather, the medical assistant says, "I really enjoy this time of year. This weather is great for exercising outdoors!"

- In the examination room, the patient mentions that she's been experiencing headaches and other symptoms for the past five days. The medical assistant nods and asks, "Could you please describe your other symptoms?"

By providing positive feedback, you'll help patients feel more comfortable discussing their private medical concerns.

so that every situation can be handled appropriately and effectively.

- Let patients and coworkers know that you respect their points of view. You can do this simply by listening attentively to what a patient or coworker has to say.
- Use good reasoning skills and persuasion in all your interactions with people.
- Emphasize to patients the need for independence. This helps build their self-concept and self-esteem.
- Encourage patients and coworkers to evaluate their own behavior. When each person takes responsibility for his own actions, it contributes to a positive work atmosphere.
- Foster an atmosphere of acceptance. Use your therapeutic communication skills to let patients and coworkers know that you accept them.
- Be sincere and genuine. Seek out role models who display respect and understanding to other people in a competent and realistic way.

Say it Isn't So

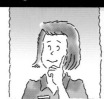

I'M NOT HAPPY AT WORK!

What should you do if you're not happy in your work environment?

The first step in improving your work environment is to make sure you're taking care of all the parts of *you*. It's more difficult for your coworkers to feel good about themselves if you're always unhappy or tired or if you have a consistently negative attitude at work. So, make sure you're following the multidimensional approach to be the best you can be physically, emotionally, mentally, and socially.

The next step is to start building the positive atmosphere you need to maintain a healthy self-concept. For example, be respectful and accepting of your coworkers. If a conflict arises, use good reasoning skills and encourage people to talk about and work out their differences. By using your therapeutic communication skills, you'll be on your way to creating a more pleasant and positive work environment.

Maslow's Hierarchy of Needs

Before you can take responsibility for your environment and well-being, you must first meet certain basic needs. This is the basis behind Abraham Maslow's **hierarchy of needs**. Maslow, an American psychologist, developed a pyramid of human needs to show how these needs are related to one another. Basic needs are at the bottom of the pyramid. Higher-level needs are at the top. Maslow suggests that people in all cultures have the same basic needs. According to Maslow's theory, lower-level needs must be met before an individual can concentrate on higher-level needs.

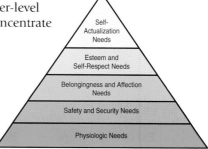

In Maslow's pyramid of human needs, lower-level needs appear at the bottom and higher-level needs appear at the top.

WHERE ARE YOU ON THE HIERARCHY?

As a medical assistant, you must be able to determine whether patients are meeting their own needs. A patient must be able to meet his basic needs before he can take responsibility for his own health. Using Maslow's hierarchy of needs will help you identify which needs a patient has or has not met.

Survival

At the bottom of the hierarchy pyramid are the most basic needs—the survival needs. These include air, water, food, rest, and shelter. If a person is unable to fulfill these basic needs, he can't begin to improve his self-image or self-esteem.

When working with patients, it's critical that you determine first if these basic needs are being met. You should also remember that the exact nature of these basic needs is different for different people. Therefore, if a patient feels that her basic needs are being met, it's important that you accept this. Be careful not to compare what others feel their basic needs are with what you feel basic needs should be.

For example, a patient may not eat meat because she is a vegetarian. You may or may not think that being a vegetarian is a good idea. But it's important that you recognize and accept that the patient feels she is fulfilling her basic diet needs. This step is required before you can effectively communicate with and help the patient.

Safety

The next level up in the hierarchy of needs includes safety needs. These are things that keep you from feeling fearful or anxious. A serious medical condition, trauma, or any sort of crisis threatens your safety needs.

After a trauma or crisis occurs, it might take time to regain a feeling of safety. You may go through a period in which you focus only on meeting your safety needs. Once your safety needs are re-established, you can move up to focus on higher needs, like love and a sense of belonging.

Love and Sense of Belonging

The third level in the hierarchy of needs includes needs for love and a sense of belonging. Fulfilling these needs helps you feel connected and important to others. These are powerful needs. They can often give you the motivation to establish or re-establish other needs.

For instance, if you have just been told you have a serious medical condition, the love of those around you may provide the incentive you need to get well. Having the desire to be healthy and stay healthy is often closely connected to the feelings you have for your loved ones.

Esteem

Your esteem needs are the needs to feel valuable and important. These needs can be fulfilled from within yourself, or they can be met by your "significant" people in your life. When other people value you, or if you value yourself, you are more likely to do what's necessary to stay in good health.

When you lack self-esteem, it's harder to *want* to learn how to get better. Learning how to improve yourself means that you care about who you are in the first place!

Self-Actualization

This is the highest level of Maslow's hierarchy pyramid. The need for self-actualization is the need to have a sense of purpose in your life. **Self-actualization** is the state of mind in which you take *full* responsibility for your health. You can only take care of this need if all your other basic needs are satisfied. It means that you do all that you can to stay healthy and happy. A self-actualized person may even help others learn to be healthier as well.

It's important to know that not all people reach this level. You, the medical assistant, must first determine where a patient is on the pyramid. If the patient's basic survival needs have not been met, you must focus on those first. Encourage the patient's "significant" people to get involved. Help the patient to realize when certain needs have been met. This will strengthen both the patient's and your own self-image and sense of accomplishment.

Listen to This   MASLOW'S HIERARCHY OF NEEDS

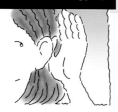

- survival needs—the need for air, water, food, rest, and shelter
- safety needs—the need to keep from feeling fearful or anxious
- love needs—the need for love and a sense of belonging
- esteem needs—the need to see yourself as a valuable person
- self-actualization needs—the need for a sense of purpose or meaning in your life

MASLOW'S HIERARCHY AND PATIENTS

Maslow's hierarchy pyramid is a helpful tool to use when you interact with patients. Whether patients will follow a plan of treatment will depend on where they are on the hierarchy pyramid. Until a patient's basic survival needs are being met, it may be impossible to expect him to follow a particular plan of treatment.

For example, suppose an elderly patient tells you that he hasn't been eating regular meals because he has a hard time getting to the grocery store. His health is suffering due to his lack of proper nutrition. To help this patient meet his basic needs, you might gather information about local organizations that provide meals. By researching and becoming familiar with community resources, you can help patients find ways of meeting their basic needs. After these basic needs are being met, the patient may be more willing to consider his other health needs and follow the physician's treatment plan.

Similarly, a patient whose love and belonging needs are not being met may be unable to focus on maintaining his health. If you encounter a patient who seems to be suffering emotionally, you may need to ask more in-depth questions, such as whether or not the patient has any family or close friends to turn to. If you note that the patient seems very distressed, your responsibility involves alerting the physician to the situation.

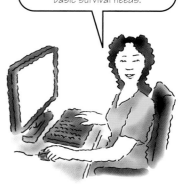

The Internet is a great place to begin your search for community resources. Local organizations, such as shelters or soup kitchens, may benefit patients who are unable to meet their basic survival needs.

The physician may recommend counseling for patients who are struggling to meet their love and belonging needs.

Developing Skills for Professional and Personal Growth

To achieve success and grow both personally and professionally, the first person that you have to please is yourself. As you have learned in this chapter, pleasing yourself means being comfortable with who you are. Also, you must be aware of your strengths and your weaknesses. There will always be someone who seems smarter, better-looking, wealthier, or more talented. Knowing this will either limit you or motivate you. But it's your choice! You need to THINK about who you are and the impact that you have on others.

T.H.I.N.K.

T.H.I.N.K. is a helpful acronym to use to help you interact with others in the most effective way possible.

- Trust your inner voice. Great potential lives inside you. To accomplish great things, you need to believe in yourself.
- Have a positive attitude. Strive to be successful. Believe that you're capable of achieving your goals and dreams.
- Inquire, then listen. There is a lot to discover. By asking questions and listening to the answers, you'll learn about yourself, about others, and about the world around you.
- Negotiate and compromise. Negotiation and compromise are often the building blocks of developing relationships.
- Know the value of kindness. Never underestimate the impact that you may have on another person's life. Treat all people with whom you interact with dignity and respect.

THE 7 HABITS OF HIGHLY EFFECTIVE PEOPLE

Another helpful tool is the popular book *The 7 Habits of Highly Effective People*. In it, well-known author Dr. Stephen Covey describes seven principles of human effectiveness. Dr. Covey believes that these are the seven primary principles on which effectiveness and happiness are based. The book encourages you to use these principles in your daily life. By doing so, he writes, you'll become a more effective professional. (You can find more information about these principles in Dr. Stephen Covey's book, *The 7 Habits of Highly Effective People.*)

Developing Insight

As you have learned, gaining insight into yourself is an important part of learning how to interact effectively with others. This is especially important when interacting with patients. You gain insight into yourself by using two types of skills—interpersonal skills and therapeutic communication skills.

INTERPERSONAL SKILLS

There are many interpersonal skills that will help you have effective interactions with patients, such as:

- *Warmth and friendliness.* Establish a warm and friendly atmosphere. This is the first step in making another person comfortable. This can be accomplished with something as simple as a warm greeting. You may not feel warm and friendly each and every day, but you can still get in the habit of behaving this way outwardly!
- *Openness and respect.* Talk and listen to others with an open mind. Listening without judging helps others feel more comfortable.
- *Empathy.* As you learned earlier in this chapter, empathy means being able to identify with another person's feelings. As a medical assistant, it's important to be able to empathize *and* still be able to help a patient work through any problems they might have.
- *Honesty, authenticity, and trust.* Always be sincere and honest. This helps patients feel comfortable enough to trust what you say and do.
- *Caring.* Let patients know that you care sincerely about them. Use your other interpersonal skills to show that you genuinely care.
- *Competence.* As a medical assistant, you have a responsibility to study and learn certain medical skills. Knowing and using these skills with confidence assures patients that they can place their trust in you.

THERAPEUTIC COMMUNICATION SKILLS

When you help patients as a medical assistant, you become involved in a relationship with these patients. But your relationship with patients is effective only when certain skills are used. Your therapeutic communication skills increase the effectiveness of this relationship.

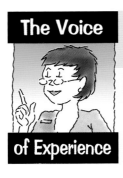

The Voice of Experience

GUIDING PRINCIPLES OF THERAPEUTIC COMMUNICATION

Q: *What does it mean to remain professional in all relationships with patients? How do I know what is professional and what is not?*

A: Remaining professional means never forgetting that you have a responsibility to the patient, the physician, and your employer. Even if the patient wants to discuss topics that do not relate to his care, such as rumor or gossip, your responsibility is to be polite, but professional, and always try to guide the conversation back to the topic of your patient's health.

Effective relationships with patients share three basic characteristics.

- They are dynamic. Both you and your patient are active participants.
- They are purposeful and time limited. You and your patient have specific goals that need to be met within a certain time period.
- The helping person is professional. You're responsible for your actions in a helping relationship; it's important to remember to present your helping abilities honestly and not to promise more than you can reasonably offer.

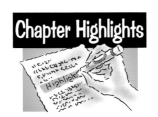

Chapter Highlights

- Self-concept is the mental image or picture you have of yourself.
- Your feelings about your personal worth can influence who you are and what you can become. If you have a positive self-concept, you'll believe in your ability to succeed.
- By assessing your strengths and weaknesses, you can continue to develop your concept of your true self.
- Feedback refers to the responses and reactions you receive from other people for your actions.
- Self-concept is a circular effect. The feedback you receive from others influences your future behavior and the way you see or feel about yourself.

- The ways you express yourself (through verbal and nonverbal messages) affect the feelings of others. For this reason, it's critical that your verbal and nonverbal messages complement each other.

- To create an atmosphere that builds self-esteem, people must treat each other with respect, be accepting of one another, and evaluate and take responsibility for their own behavior.

- Take a multidimensional approach to building the physical, mental, psychological, and social characteristics that will help you achieve a positive self-image. Ask yourself questions such as, "Am I getting enough exercise?" and "Do I get together with friends often?"

- Maslow's hierarchy includes human needs related to survival, safety, love and belonging, esteem, and self-actualization.

- To communicate more effectively, develop interpersonal skills, such as friendliness, empathy, and respect. Use therapeutic communication techniques to establish a helping relationship with the patients you care for.

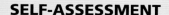

Active Learning

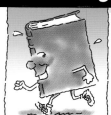

SELF-ASSESSMENT

On your own, take an honest look at your strengths and weaknesses. List your strengths, being sure to include physical, emotional, and social characteristics. Then, think about your weaknesses. In what areas of your life do you find yourself struggling? Think about the talents, knowledge, or abilities that could help you function more effectively at your job. Come up with a plan for turning each of your weaknesses into strengths.

Group Discussion: Role Models

Divide into groups of three or four and take turns describing a role model in your life. Discuss your role model's impact and influence on the person you have become.

Chapter 2

THE COMMUNICATION CYCLE

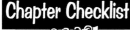

Chapter Checklist

- Discuss the importance of communication

- Describe the communication cycle

- Define *message, channel of communication, receiver, sender,* and *feedback*

- Demonstrate understanding of the difference between verbal and nonverbal messages

- Discuss the impact of tone of voice, choice of words, and body posture on communication

- State the importance of developing listening skills

- Discuss the difference between social and therapeutic communication

- Demonstrate understanding of therapeutic and nontherapeutic communication techniques

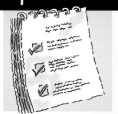

Chapter Competencies

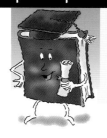

- Be attentive, listen, and learn (ABHES Competency 2.a.)

- Be impartial and show empathy when dealing with patients (ABHES Competency 2.b.)

- Recognize and respond to verbal and nonverbal communication (ABHES Competency 2.i., 2.k., and 2.l.; CAAHEP Competency 3.c.1.b. and 3.c.3.c.)

Take a moment to think about how you communicate with people. Have you ever thought about the signals you give to others as you chat with friends, discuss assignments with instructors, or give presentations to fellow students? As a medical assistant, you'll exchange information with physicians, other medical assistants, patients, and office personnel. You need to be able to communicate this information effectively and appropriately. Often, one of the first people a patient encounters in the medical office is a medical assistant. Therefore, the quality of this first experience may set the tone for all the patient's future visits to the office.

In this chapter, you'll learn about the elements of the communication cycle and the different types of communication that we use to relay our message. You'll discover the importance of listening. This chapter will also show you ways you can apply therapeutic communication skills to your day-to-day interactions with patients.

Communication: It's More than Just Talking

People share information by communicating. Although the way people do this may differ, the basic nature of all communication is the same—information is shared.

When you arrive at work in the morning, you may share information about how you're feeling, how your evening was the night before, or what you did that morning. The people you work with may do the same. As the day goes on, you share many kinds of information with coworkers as well as with patients.

Sharing information by chatting with coworkers isn't the only way you receive or give information. Every time you read a magazine, newspaper, letter, or even a bill, information is being shared. When you offer a lending hand to someone, smile pleasantly, give an encouraging look, or simply touch a patient's shoulder to comfort him, you're sharing information.

THE IMPORTANCE OF COMMUNICATION

People have always relied on some system of communication to share information. Early humans used pictures and simple sounds. Over time, people have developed different languages to communicate with each other. Hand gestures and facial expressions can also be used to communicate.

When you communicate with patients, your basic goal is to share information. Being able to do this effectively makes you a better caregiver. Learning to know how and when to communicate with patients takes time. There are many signals and clues that you can learn to observe in a patient. Knowing these will help you to communicate effectively and appropriately with any patient in any situation.

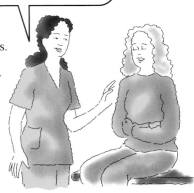

Is there anything I can do to help you feel more comfortable? Would you like a glass of water?

For example, a patient may feel uncomfortable or embarrassed about her illness. She may be very quiet and withdrawn and only offer short, one-word responses to your questions. How you respond to the patient's signals—what you say to her and how you say it—can make her feel less uncomfortable and more at ease. As a result, the patient's experience becomes more positive. Over time, she may feel more comfortable and be more likely to share important details of her illness that you and the physician need to know to provide her with the best possible care.

WHY EFFECTIVE COMMUNICATION HELPS

Effective communication is important not just in medical assisting, but in all kinds of professional positions. In a survey of managers, communication skills and the ability to get along with others were listed as the two most important factors in choosing a new manager. Learning effective communication helps your patients and your career.

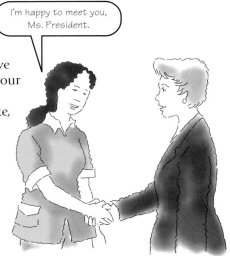

I'm happy to meet you, Ms. President.

An effective communicator is able to write, speak, listen, and respond in the right way at the right time. Learning these skills is a critical part of your role as a medical assistant. The more you practice good communication skills, the more comfortable you'll be when interacting with people from all backgrounds. This will help you not only in your career as a medical assistant, but in your personal life, too!

COMMUNICATION BREAKDOWN

Sometimes, you may not be as successful in the way you communicate with others as you would like. If your communication breaks down, you may find it more difficult to achieve your goals. Here are some scenarios that show communication breakdowns.

- You send an e-mail you think is funny to your supervisor, but she finds your e-mail offensive.
- You're nervous drawing a patient's blood for the first time, and he senses you're not confident.
- You're up late with a sick family member and keep yawning during class the next day until your instructor asks if she is boring you.

You need to be prepared for communication breakdowns like those listed above. More importantly, you should know how to avoid them. Remember that what you say is as important as how you say it. You should always be aware of your facial expressions and consider how others might interpret your actions.

In addition, increasing importance is placed on developing both written and oral communication skills as computers and e-mails replace face-to-face interactions. Individuals who are unable to communicate effectively are at a distinct disadvantage in the workplace. Lacking these communication skills may prove to be a major roadblock as you work to move ahead in your career.

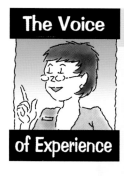

The Voice of Experience

IS SHE RUDE, OR AM I TOO SENSITIVE?

Q: *There is a coworker in my office who constantly makes fun of patients. She comments on patients' ages, their hairstyles, and their clothing choices, and she makes faces if they have body odor. I am uncomfortable with the way she acts, but she only does it when the patients can't see or hear her. Am I overreacting?*

A: You're definitely not overreacting. The way your coworker responds to patients is rude and possibly unethical. It may seem that the coworker is not doing any harm, because the patients can't hear her rude comments, but communication does not come from just words. If your coworker thinks poorly of patients in general, she is less likely to treat them with respect. She may not smile at them or try to put them at ease while they are waiting for the physician. She may not provide support, encouragement, or additional information if a patient needs assistance after receiving a difficult diagnosis.

You should first try to speak to your coworker and remind her of her ethical obligations to patients. If that does not work, you may need to speak to your supervisor about it.

The Communication Cycle

Suppose a physician is going to remove some sutures from a patient's arm. You're interviewing the patient prior to the procedure. You need to find out if the patient has experienced any redness or swelling while the sutures have been in place. So, what is the best way to get this information from the patient? How do you know that the patient understands what you have asked him?

To answer these questions, you must first understand the parts of the communication cycle. The communication cycle includes a message, a receiver, a sender, and feedback.

THE MESSAGE

A **message** is any thought or idea that is sent to another person. You send messages to patients, coworkers, family, and friends. You may not think about it, but you even send messages to strangers.

The Quality of a Message

Several factors affect the quality of a message.

- Your *tone* when sending a message should show interest, not boredom. The messages you send to patients should always be sincere and genuine. In the example above, your tone in explaining the suture removal procedure to the patient should be calm, factual, and reassuring.

- *What is being communicated* in the message affects how you send the message. Discussing a sensitive issue with a patient requires patience and understanding on your part. In the example, you want to assure the patient about the safety of the procedure, what will happen during the procedure, and the purpose of the procedure.

- *What is left out* of a message can send critical nonverbal messages. Asking a patient everything except how he is feeling would be confusing, since patients expect that you're concerned about how they feel.

- Your *individual style* of communicating makes your messages unique to you. All of your verbal and nonverbal communication skills add spark and color to your messages. Going back to the example, your ability to inform and reassure the patient depends on the communication skills you have learned and mastered!

Channels of Communication

When you think of ways you send messages to others, you probably think of speaking, listening, using body gestures, body language, or writing. But messages can be shared in other ways, too. The meaning of your message is often determined by the way you send it. For example, a sentence spoken out loud may be interpreted differently if it were sent in an e-mail. Also, feelings such as sadness, disappointment, anger, or confusion are sometimes more difficult to get across in written messages. The different ways that you can send a message are called *channels of communication.*

Here are some examples of channels of communication:

- Face-to-face meetings allow you to share not only the words you speak, but also your body language and facial expressions. Face-to-face meetings are often the best way to communicate very sensitive information, such as a frightening diagnosis.

- Phone conversations are a convenient way to send messages with people who are far away, busy at work, or simply not available for a face-to-face conversation. Without the ability to see facial expressions or body language, however, it can be difficult to share sensitive or personal information over the phone.

- Video conferences allow several people to communicate with one another without being in the same room. Computer monitors are used so that each person involved in the conference can see the others' faces. Microphones or speakers are used so that the members of the conference can hear what everyone is saying.

- Webcasting allows you or a group of people to communicate with many people on the World Wide Web. A Webcast is like a video diary that's shown on the Internet. This is a good way to share information with a large group of people in a short period of time.

- Written forms like letters, e-mails, memos, faxes, and reports are good ways to send business or personal messages to others. Again, it's difficult to get across emotions in written form. Some people are better at it than others.

- Text messaging allows you to send and receive written messages with a cellular phone. This is a good method for communicating very brief messages.

SENDER

The person who sends the first message in a communication is the **sender.** Because the sender starts the communication, there is considerable responsibility placed on the sender's shoulders. The sender must decide:

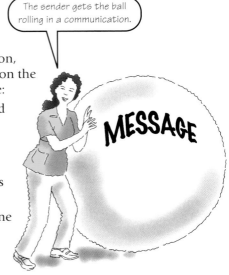

The sender gets the ball rolling in a communication.

- what form the communication should take
- when to communicate
- what words to use in the message
- what body language or which gestures to use

The sender is responsible for setting the tone of the communication and sending a clear message.

RECEIVER

The person who receives the sender's message is the **receiver.** If you're the receiver, you decode and interpret the message sent by the sender. Remember, the sender starts the ball rolling in a communication. But the receiver is the one who catches the ball.

Have you ever said or written something to somebody that was misunderstood? As the receiver, your job is to decode the message and to figure out what the sender's message means.

FEEDBACK

Feedback is the way that a receiver responds to the message. The receiver might be overjoyed, hurt, surprised, disappointed, pleased, or offended by the sender's message. The receiver's feedback may be verbal or nonverbal.

Effective feedback lets the sender know if the message was interpreted and understood by the receiver. Ineffective feedback does not let the sender know how the message was interpreted and understood.

Think again about the how the sender starts the ball rolling, passing it along to the receiver. The feedback happens when the receiver gets the ball and announces to the sender, "I got it!"

Positive Feedback

Positive feedback lets the sender know that the message was received positively. Here are some examples of positive feedback:

- A soothing message might be received with a smile.
- A funny message might be received with a laugh or a chuckle.
- A surprising message might be received with a gasp.

Whatever the case, positive feedback lets the sender know that the message was received in a good way.

Negative Feedback

Negative feedback can also be an effective way to respond to a message. Let's go back to the message ball. If the sender throws the ball too hard to the receiver, the receiver might get hurt and yell in pain. Even though the receiver wasn't happy with the message, at least the sender knows he received it! Negative feedback tells the sender that the message was hurtful in some way.

It's good to remember that negative feedback is not always a bad thing. Consider this example. You ask your supervisor how you're doing at a new task, and he says that you still need some practice. His feedback is negative, but it's not ineffective. Even though you might have received news you didn't want to hear, you have confirmed that your receiver got your message and interpreted it correctly.

Context: The What, Where, When, and How of Communication

The situation, or **context**, in which messages are delivered and received influences the outcome of any communication. For instance, suppose you have an urgent personal message to deliver to a coworker. You see the coworker rushing down the hallway on the other side of the building. Yelling the message to the coworker would be an ineffective way of delivering this message.

It's important for you as the participant in a communication to help create the right situation for the communication to take place. For example, a personal message should be delivered so that only the receiver hears or reads it. This is especially important in the medical office when communicating private information with the patient, physician, or coworkers.

A handy tool to keep in mind when communicating with others is the five Cs of communication. The five Cs are five easy ways to help guarantee the proper context of your communication with others.

To create the right context for communication, the message must be:

- Clear—make sure the message is easy to understand. Speak carefully and clearly. Written messages should be easy to read and understand.
- Culturally sensitive—messages should take into consideration a person's cultural beliefs, practices, and values.
- Complete—messages should contain all information that is necessary. Do not leave out important details.
- Courteous—messages should be delivered in a courteous manner. Be considerate of others' feelings and time.
- Consistent—messages must be organized and rational. Sometimes it helps to think about what you need to say before you say it. Read written messages before you send them.

To Speak or Not to Speak—Verbal and Nonverbal Communication

The majority of your communication happens when you're face-to-face with another person. Some of your messages might be spoken, or verbal. Others might be nonspoken, or nonverbal. Both verbal and nonverbal forms of communication are effective when used in the right way at the right time.

VERBAL COMMUNICATION

Verbal communication means sending and receiving messages using spoken language. As a medical assistant, you'll speak with patients, coworkers, and physicians on a daily basis. As a professional, you should always use proper English and grammar. In verbal communication, *how* something is said is often as important as *what* is said. Here are some of the elements of effective verbal communication.

Voice Quality

The quality of your voice helps determine how your messages are received. A soothing voice is comforting. A harsh voice may make a receiver uncomfortable. Make sure the quality of your voice fits the kind of message you want to send. For example, if you're taking a patient's blood pressure, your voice should be calm and soothing.

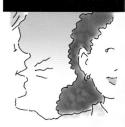

Send and Receive

USING THE FIVE Cs OF COMMUNICATION

How can using the five Cs of communication help you as a medical assistant? Here is an example that shows how the five Cs can make a difference in the way you communicate with patients.

Ineffective:

- The medical assistant is rushed and speeds through her instructions to the patient. "Here you go, Mr. Alder. Call us in two weeks for a follow-up. Take these tablets for your pain. I do not know why the physician gave you tablets instead of capsules. I prefer the capsules myself. The directions are on the bottle."
- "Have a good day, Mr. Alder."
- "Oh wait, I forgot to give you your tablets! Here."
- "Oh and do not forget to make an appointment in 10 days . . . or was it 2 weeks? Let me check. Yes, it's 2 weeks. So, okay, take your capsules . . . I mean, tablets. Bye."

Patients can be confused or frightened when they come to a physician's office. It's important to follow the five Cs when you interact with them. This means taking a little extra time to explain things, speaking more slowly, recognizing any cultural preferences, and asking the patient if they have any questions.

Effective:

- The medical assistant takes her time with the patient. "Here you go, Mr. Alder. Take one of these pills every 12 hours until they're gone. The physician prescribed tablets instead of capsules because the dosage you need comes only in tablet form. If you begin to experience any side effects, be sure to call us."
- "Let's go up to the front desk on your way out, and we'll make an appointment for 2 weeks from now."
- "Do you have any questions?"

This time, the medical assistant makes sure the patient is following what she is telling him. She does this by speaking *clearly* in a *courteous* manner. Her instructions to the patient are *culturally sensitive, complete,* and *consistent.* Also, she asks the patient if he has any questions. In other words, the sender asks the receiver for feedback to make sure the messages were effectively communicated.

Intention

The purpose of your message is your intention. Your intention is reflected in the way you phrase your message. For instance, before you take a patient's blood pressure you might say, "All right, Mrs. Brown, I'm going to take your blood pressure now. Can you put your arm out for me?" You wouldn't command, "Give me your arm." This would confuse the patient—and probably raise her blood pressure!

Manner

Manner is the way a message is presented. Speaking gently, directly, and sincerely to patients lets them know that you care. It's important that your intention and manner match. Your manner in addressing patients should be nonthreatening and reassuring. This tells them that you're about to do something that will help.

Maintaining eye contact is important, but too much can turn a good thing bad. Look relaxed, not intense!

Eye Contact

Looking directly at a patient lets her know that you're focused on her. Sending a message without looking at the receiver is confusing. The receiver might think you do not really want to talk to him. Patients might think you'd rather be somewhere else. Making and maintaining eye contact when you speak sends a positive message. It helps build trust and honesty between you and the receiver.

Self-Concept

People can tell how you feel about yourself by listening to the way you use your voice. A confident self-concept comes through the confidence in your voice. When you tell Mrs. Brown that you're about to take her blood pressure, you should do it with confidence—"Mrs. Brown, I'm going to take your blood pressure now." Mrs. Brown might think twice about letting you take her blood pressure if you say, "Uh, Mrs. Brown, I'm, uh, I mean I'm going to try to, uh, take your, uh, blood pressure. Now let me see if I remember how to do this." If you hesitate or doubt your abilities, the patient will sense it.

Setting: Time, Place, and Timing

Where you are, the time of day, and the timing of your conversation with others affects the efficiency of the communication. Would you try to take Mrs. Brown's blood pressure outside the office on the sidewalk? At 10 o'clock at night? Would you tell

Mrs. Brown about your sick cat while you take her blood pressure? Of course not!

You should also remember that certain topics might require more thought as to the time, place, and setting of a conversation. Discussing diet concerns with a patient recently diagnosed with diabetes will take longer than a standard appointment. This discussion should take place in the physician's office and not while the patient is on her way out the door. Your spoken messages will be received best when they are sent in the appropriate setting, time, place, and with the proper timing.

Sensitivity

For some people, certain topics might be difficult to talk about. Part of your job as a medical assistant is to know whether the person you're talking to may be sensitive about certain subjects. When sensitive subjects must be discussed, take extra care in your tone and manner, maintain eye contact, and choose the appropriate setting, time, and place.

Attitude and Confidence

Your overall attitude and level of confidence comes through your spoken words. Like your positive self-concept, a positive attitude and strong level of confidence help to make your communications more effective. An insecure person can show his insecurity by speaking quietly, by shouting, or by being "tough." In contrast, a person who speaks with confidence speaks aloud without shouting or talking over others.

NONVERBAL COMMUNICATION

What you do not say often has a bigger impact on your receiver than what you do say. Some studies have shown that for most interactions, the actual words you use make up only a small percentage of the total message your receiver receives. Tone of voice makes up another small percentage of the message. It might surprise you to know that nonverbal cues (like facial expressions, hand gestures, and posture) make up nearly 70% of your total message!

Nonverbal cues play the biggest role in making communication effective. Here are some of the ways you communicate nonverbally with others.

Facial Expressions

Facial expressions send many kinds of nonverbal messages. The face is the most expressive part of the body. Without saying a single word, you let people know when you're sad, angry,

Listen to This

COMMUNICATING VERBALLY WITH PATIENTS

In order to provide the best care to patients, you'll need to develop excellent verbal communication skills. You might be surprised at how much information you can get from a patient about her condition just by asking the right questions.

Here are six things that will help you conduct effective interviews. These methods also can be used in other settings to improve communication.

- *Restate.* Repeat part of what you hear the person say and let him finish the sentence. For example, "You were saying that your back hurts you when you . . ." Restating encourages people to give you more information.

- *Paraphrase.* Repeat what you've heard using your own words or phrases. Paraphrasing is a way of making sure you understood what was said. It usually begins by saying, "You're saying that . . ." or "It sounds as if . . ." followed by your best explanation of what your patient has told you.

- *Clarify.* Ask for examples when a patient gives you information that's confusing or hard to understand. For instance, ask, "Can you describe one of those dizzy spells?" The patient's example should help you better understand what he's saying.

- *Ask open-ended questions.* Ask questions in ways that can't be answered with just a yes or a no. Begin questions with what, when, how, and why. When asking why questions—such as, "Why did you stop taking your medicine?"—be sure that your tone is not judgmental.

- *Summarize.* Briefly review the information you have gathered. This gives the patient a chance to correct wrong or unclear information. For example, suppose a patient reports stumbling often. You might summarize by saying, "You told me that you've been feeling dizzy and that you often stumble as you walk."

- *Allow silence.* Allow periods of silence. Silences can encourage people to talk more. Some people are uncomfortable with pauses in conversations. They feel the need to fill the silence with words. Silences also can be used to think about what's already been said.

scared, suspicious, or joyful. A simple, friendly "hello" seems angry if you deliver it with a grimace on your face.

It's important that you, as a professional, learn to control your own facial expressions. As a medical assistant, you'll be in many situations when you might want to react to a patient's wound or condition with an inappropriate facial expression. To do so, however, would affect the patient's self-concept and recovery in a negative way. Make sure your facial expressions are appropriate for the situation. Consider the patient's well-being and self-concept at all times.

Vocal Paralanguage

Research has shown that the meaning of a message is determined more by the way a message is sent than by the words in the message itself. Clues in your voice add meaning and emphasis to your messages. These extra clues are called your **vocal paralanguage.** They include tone, quality, volume, pitch, and range. The simple "hello" greeting would be received very differently if it were delivered with a harsh tone, loud volume, and high pitch.

A point to remember is how your vocal paralanguage affects the way a receiver interprets your messages. Be aware of the kind of feedback you get from a receiver. If the feedback is not what you expected, perhaps your vocal paralanguage was at fault.

Hand Gestures

The way you use or do not use your hands to send a message can help or hurt the way that message is received and interpreted. Let's go back to offering the simple "hello" message. Suppose you deliver the "hello" greeting with your arms crossed and your fists clenched. The receiver might interpret your greeting as insincere or unfriendly. In contrast, a quick wave combined with a friendly "hello" results in a more genuine greeting.

Kinesics

The way you use your body when you send messages can also be critical. Your **kinesics,** or body movements, have a strong effect on the messages you send to others. As a medical assistant, your patients should feel that you're sincere and committed to helping them. The kinesics you use with patients should show these qualities.

When you're preparing to interview a patient, take a moment to check that your stance is open. This means that:

- you're facing the patient
- your expression shows you're interested
- your legs and arms are relaxed and comfortable

While you speak to the patient, stay calm and controlled. Relax your arms and legs. Remind yourself to show a kind and friendly expression on your face. This will show the patient that you're genuinely interested in helping him.

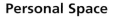

If you uncross your arms, you'll feel more open—and patients will interpret your message positively!

Touch

Touch is one of the most effective nonverbal forms of communication. For example, placing your hand on a patient's shoulder may send an invaluable message of comfort and support to a patient who is fearful and upset. However, it's important to remember that not all patients will react the same way to a gentle touch. Patients may react to touch differently based on their culture, family background, region, age, or sex. Consider each patient as an individual before offering a comforting pat on the shoulder.

Personal Space

Every person has a comfortable distance that they maintain between themselves and others. For most patients this **personal space** is a distance of 18 inches to 48 inches. As a medical assistant, you'll often need to get close to patients when performing certain tasks. In general, you should stand close enough to patients to make them feel comfortable and not threatened. Consider any feedback you receive from patients. If a patient seems uncomfortable during an interview, perhaps you're sitting too close. If a patient seems distracted, perhaps you're sitting too far away.

Posture

Your posture is part of your kinesics, which was discussed earlier. But your posture while moving and standing is an important part of your nonverbal communication. The way you carry your body affects the messages you send to others. A receiver interprets the content of your message along with the posture you have when you deliver the message.

Earlier in this chapter you read using an open stance to send a message of genuine interest, respect, and empathy. Sending a message with an open stance means standing or sitting facing toward another person. Your legs should be comfortably apart and arms uncrossed. Your facial expression should be kind and friendly.

Territoriality

Your urge to claim certain spaces as your own is **territoriality**. The patients you see in the office would probably act differently if you saw them in their own homes. Likewise, you probably do and say things differently in your own home than you do at work. As a medical assistant, it's important to understand how territoriality affects your interactions with patients. Always behave professionally when you're at work. Let your patients know, by your actions and your words, that you're knowledgeable, confident, and capable.

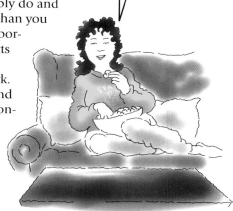

Because of territoriality, you send different messages when you're at home than when you're at work.

CONGRUENT AND INCONGRUENT MESSAGES

From time to time, a verbal message and a nonverbal message may not match. When this happens, the receiver becomes

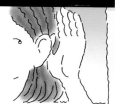

Listen to This

KEYS TO NONVERBAL COMMUNICATION

Here are some guidelines for getting the most out of nonverbal communications:

1. Maintain proper personal space, position, and posture. Your nonverbal communication is sending messages to the patient, too.
   - Always look the patient in the face and be at eye level. Be aware of cultural differences when it comes to eye contact.
   - If the patient is sitting, you should sit, too.
   - Use proper gestures.
   - Use touch, if the situation is appropriate.

2. Observe the patient's facial expressions and posture. People's nonverbal messages can differ from their verbal ones.
   - If the patient's nonverbal clues differ from what he is saying, ask appropriate questions to clarify the mixed message.
   - If a patient's verbal response does not match what you're seeing, document your observations and share your concerns with the physician.

confused. The way that a message is sent—the process—and what the message contains—the content—should agree.

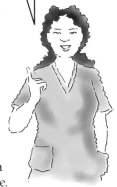

Here's a good communication goal to set for yourself: all messages that you send should be congruent messages.

Congruent Message

In a **congruent message**, the content and process of the message agree. For example, your verbal message to a patient might be, "I'd really like to help you." Similarly, your body language and gestures also let the patient know that help is being offered. You might offer your hand to help the patient get up from an exam table. As a result, the patient knows and understands the meaning of your message.

Incongruent Message

In an **incongruent message**, the content and process of the message disagree. For example, your verbal message might be "I'd really like to help you." But your nonverbal message might include no eye contact and a closed stance. This sends a message to the patient that you do not really want to help at all. As a result, the receiver is confused about the meaning of the message.

Listening

Having good listening skills is critical for good communication. Learning how to actively listen will help you with all of your interpersonal interactions. An active listener paraphrases the sender's message to make sure it was interpreted correctly. There are several elements of good listening.

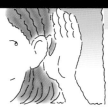

Listen to This

CONGRUENT AND INCONGRUENT MESSAGES

Here are a few examples of incongruent messages:

- You have had a busy, tiring day at work. You've just been asked to work an extra hour. You respond by grumbling "Oh sure, no problem."
- A patient hangs her head and looks down. You ask her how she is feeling. She sighs and says, "I'm fine."
- A coworker has been snapping at people all day. You finally ask her if there's anything you can do to help. She snaps back, "I do not need any help!"

ELEMENTS OF LISTENING

Trying to understand a patient's thoughts and feelings is a critical part of your job as a medical assistant. But it's not always easy! This chapter has talked a lot about how to send messages effectively. But what about listening? Being able to listen effectively to what others say to you is just as important as speaking effectively. There are many ways that you can sharpen your listening skills.

Be Attentive

Use body language and gestures to let the person know you're listening. Use the open stance. Face the speaker. Everything about your posture and body language should tell the speaker that you're paying attention.

Make Eye Contact

Make eye contact with the person speaking to you. Do not allow yourself to look away, unless you're doing so temporarily to take notes. Avoiding a speaker's eyes sends a message to the speaker that you're not interested. Maintain eye contact while the speaker is talking, and you let the speaker know that you're actively listening.

Get Engaged

Engaging with the speaker means that you're letting the speaker know that you connect with her. When you're engaged, you connect with what is being said. An occasional "I see" or nodding your head lets the speaker know that you're not only paying attention, but that you understand what she is saying.

Patients respond positively when you're engaged with them. They feel that you're completely focused on helping them. Learning how to engage in all conversations helps you listen more attentively whenever you communicate.

Stay Open

Staying open lets a speaker know you're open to what is being said. Your body language, eye contact, gestures, and facial expressions show the speaker that you're interested and engaged with what is being said.

Many patients may make comments or have beliefs that you do not agree with. Remember to keep your personal opinions out of your conversations with patients. Keep an open mind as you work with patients from other cultures and countries. Be tolerant of other beliefs. If patients sense your disapproval or lack of acceptance, they will not be as willing to interact with you.

Learn Body Language

Your body language plays a big role when communicating with others. To let others know you're actively listening, always use the open stance—arms down to your side, full front, facing the other person. Make eye contact, relax your arms and legs, and make sure your expression is kind and friendly.

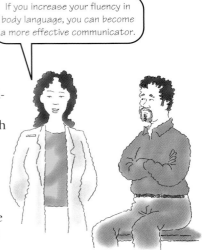

If you increase your fluency in body language, you can become a more effective communicator.

When you meet a patient for the first time, you'll need to ask a lot of questions. Understanding how to "read" other people's body language will help with this task. If a patient comes in with crossed arms and a grouchy expression, you'll have to change your approach to meet your patient's state of mind. Maybe the patient just had an argument with his spouse or is having a bad day. Or maybe the patient is just often in a bad mood. You can't always know why someone is upset, but just recognizing that he is upset can make your communication more effective.

Offer Feedback

When you're the receiver of communication, the nonverbal cues you give to the sender are feedback. The only way patients know that you understand them is from the feedback you offer. Here are some examples of feedback.

- Your nonverbal feedback could be your open stance, your constant eye contact, or your gentle gestures and expressions.
- The ways you engage a patient in conversation is also a form of feedback. During the conversation, nod, smile, or respond with an appropriate facial expression.
- When the other patient is done talking, offer a comment or two. Share your thoughts or feelings about what was said.
- Finally, ask any necessary follow-up questions.

Putting Your Communication Skills to Work

The communications you have with patients are very different than the ones you have with family or friends. Although both can be caring, trusting, and supporting interactions, there are some differences. Social communications can happen at any time. They often have no specific purpose.

On the other hand, therapeutic communications—those you have with patients—are much more specific. For example, you meet with a specific person—a patient. You have a definite purpose when you meet with a patient. The amount and type of information that is shared is different for you than it is for the patient. The patient shares personal, health-related information. You share professional care-related information. Also, therapeutic communication is usually limited by time and space. You have only a set amount of time to interact with a patient. The place where you interact is also often limited to a specific room or building.

BUILDING COMMUNICATIONS IN THE WORKPLACE

Remember, the primary purpose of your therapeutic communications is to help the patient. The way you communicate paves the way for more effective interactions between you and your patients. Here are some factors that will help increase the effectiveness of your therapeutic communications.

Confidentiality

It's your responsibility as a medical assistant to let the patient know with whom his health information will be shared. Federal law governs the release of patient information. (You'll learn more about the laws governing patient confidentiality in Chapter 4.) Remember that the patient should know about his right to say who might have access to such information. Address the patient's right to privacy by taking the time to explain this legal right to the patient.

Active Listening

When you listen actively to patients, you give them your full attention. When communicating with patients, always keep interruptions to a minimum. Be aware of the patient's vocal paralanguage, body language, and other nonverbal means of communication the patient might use.

Observation

Take care to observe everything about a patient. Observe the patient even when he is not speaking. Pay attention to how the patient listens *and* speaks. Look for clues about things the patient might not share with you verbally.

Be sure to observe yourself and how you're interacting with the patient. If you receive negative feedback from a patient, try to make any necessary corrections. If you receive positive feed-back, congratulate yourself for communicating so well!

Respect

Be respectful of the patient's personal space, time, and concerns. Under no circumstances should you ever insult, tease, or ridicule a patient. All patients, regardless of race, gender, age, culture, occupation, or religious belief, deserve your tolerance and acceptance.

Self-Disclosure

Some patients may find it difficult to share their personal information. Help patients feel more comfortable by providing them with a safe, private, supportive environment. Reassure patients using your verbal and nonverbal communication skills. Offer a warm handshake, listen attentively, and reassure them with a gentle touch.

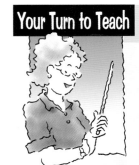

Your Turn to Teach | **ACTIVELY LISTEN**

A patient sits in the examination room with his head down, arms folded, and shoulders slouched. You must collect some basic information about the patient before the physician sees him. Practice your active listening skills by following these steps:

- The patient's body language clearly says that he is uncomfortable and not feeling well. To help the patient feel as comfortable as possible, make sure the room is private and quiet.

- Address the patient by his name. Make eye contact. Be warm, courteous, and respectful. Face the patient using an open stance. Ask questions clearly.

- Give the patient your full attention when talking *and* listening. Allow the patient to speak without interrupting.

- Be aware of how the patient communicates nonverbally. What is the patient's posture? Does the patient use hand gestures? What kinds of facial expressions does the patient have? What are the patient's kinesics, or body movements?

- Acknowledge the patient's concerns and fears. Actively listen! Pay full attention to what the patient tells you. Do not allow your thoughts to wander or distract you.

YOUR COMMUNICATION GOALS

Every time you meet with a patient, your communication with that patient should accomplish several goals. Keeping these goals in mind will help guarantee a strong relationship between you and your patients. Use these goals to review what helps make your communication skills as effective as possible.

Know Your Role

Your role as medical assistant and the patient's role as a patient should be clear from the beginning of all your interactions. Doing this will send a clear message to the patient that you're a confident, capable medical professional.

Know the Patient's Concern

Observe the patient's verbal and nonverbal messages to identify the reason for the patient's visit. Ask questions clearly and thoroughly. Collect as much information as you need to give the physician a complete picture of the patient's concern.

Know How the Patient Feels

To best help the patient, you should determine the patient's perception of the problem. Help the patient describe what he thinks the problem might be. Patients usually know themselves better than anybody else does. Allow the patient to talk freely about his concern.

Know the Patient's Needs

Recognize the patient's underlying needs and assess whether the patient's basic needs are being met. Is the patient getting enough sleep, food, and exercise? Is the patient going through any sort of personal crisis that might affect his health?

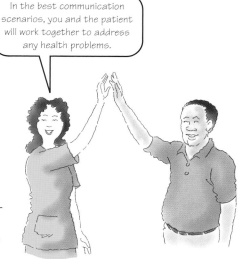

In the best communication scenarios, you and the patient will work together to address any health problems.

Know How to Help the Patient

You should always enlist the patient's support in working toward a solution. Help the patient create a strategy for treating his problem. Review each step of the strategy and then ask the patient if he has questions.

Developing Your Communication Skills

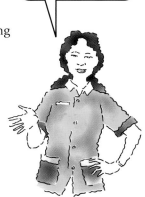

You might want to make a list of the essential communication skills and use it as a quick review once you've begun working in a medical setting.

The effectiveness of your communications with patients depends on the skills you have as a good communicator. As you gain experience in the field, you might pick up new skills that have not been discussed in this chapter. Whatever skills you collect in your communications tool bag, remember that the harder you work at communicating effectively, the better you'll be.

THERAPEUTIC COMMUNICATION TECHNIQUES

This chapter has discussed many ways that people communicate and listen to each other. How can you use this knowledge as a medical professional? Here are some essential communication skills to keep in mind when working with patients.

Ask Open-Ended Questions

An **open-ended question** is a question that can't be answered by a simple yes or no. Open-ended questions begin with "How do you feel about . . ." or "What are your reasons for thinking that . . ." Whenever possible, try to avoid asking questions that begin with why, such as "Why didn't you take your medicine?" Such questions can sound judgmental. They may make some patients feel that they have to provide an excuse or justification for their actions.

Remember that one of your responsibilities is to gather information from the patient about his concerns and needs. If your questions tend to generate one-word answers, it will be much more difficult for you to collect essential information. Open-ended questions allow patients to express how they feel in their own words.

Actively Listen

Always practice active listening! The more you practice it, the better you'll get. Here are some ways to engage in active listening.

- Remember to look directly at the patient. Maintain eye contact.
- Engage the patient. Offer feedback to let the patient know you're listening and understanding what he is saying. Remember that feedback can be verbal or nonverbal.
- If you do not understand something the patient has said, ask him to repeat or explain.

Use Broad Openings

Begin your conversation with a patient with general questions. Zero in on specific issues gradually. Patients are often nervous when they come to a physician's office. It may be difficult for them to open up and share their personal information or a specific private concern. Help them by starting out with general questions. Once you sense the patient relaxing, then you can ask more specific questions.

Use Your Nonverbal Skills

Let patients know with your gestures and body language that you're there to help and support them. Remember to use your vocal paralanguage, facial expressions, eye contact, touch, and kinesics. All of these tools will help make your messages clear and effective.

Give Feedback

Offer patients your sincere feedback to their comments. Also, make sure your own messages are clear to the patient. In short, let patients know that you understand their messages to you. This builds the patient's self-confidence and strengthens the interaction between you and the patient.

Acknowledge Feelings

Let patients know that you have sensed when they are upset, concerned, sad, uncomfortable, or angry. You can do this verbally by saying, "I see you're upset." Or, you can acknowledge nonverbally by holding the patient's hand or resting your hand on his shoulder. Acknowledging the patient's feelings lets him know you're paying attention to his needs and concerns. It also means that you're observing the patient's verbal and nonverbal messages.

NONTHERAPEUTIC TECHNIQUES

Although there may be times when nontherapeutic communication methods may appear to be useful, they should not be used with patients.

Advising Patients

Offering your own advice to a patient is unprofessional and unethical. It also imposes your personal opinions and feelings on the patient. For example, telling a patient that your personal preference for pain medication is different from what the physician has prescribed would be inappropriate. Any questions or concerns that a patient has should be carefully written down and shared with the physician.

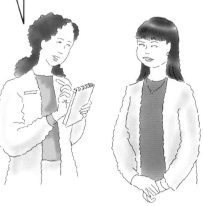

I understand your concerns. Let's talk with the physician and come to a decision together.

Defensive Responses

Patients depend on your confidence and self-assurance. You should not allow yourself to become defensive if a patient questions the plan of treatment. It may be that she is simply trying to better understand what the physician has prescribed for her. Would you say to a patient, "The doctor would never have told you that"? Of course not. That makes you sound defensive and may make the patient feel inferior. You may want explain the physician's instructions. You could also write down any questions the patient may have, and then relay them to the physician. Or, suggest to the patient that she address her questions or concerns directly with the physician.

Changing the Subject

There may be times when changing the subject of a conversation might be helpful. It's important to know when changing the subject is okay and when it's not. Listening to and observing the patient will help you decide if changing the subject is a good idea. Otherwise, it may send a message to the patient that you're bored or not interested in what he has to say.

Using Reassuring Clichés

An occasional "Hold your horses!" or "It's as easy as pie!" can lighten a conversation. But be careful to avoid relying on clichés as your sole means of communication. When used at the wrong time or too often, clichés like "Cheer up, tomorrow's another day!" get in the way of your ability to listen effectively to what a patient is trying to tell you.

Clichés can also interfere with your ability to communicate important information to a patient. Patients who speak English as a second language may not understand the intended meaning of a cliché.

Additionally, avoid using the cliché, "He's in a better place" when talking with those who have lost a loved one. This cliché may not apply to people of certain religious backgrounds. It can also be difficult for surviving friends and family members to hear and may not provide the comfort you intend.

Judging

Keep your mind open when communicating with all patients. Use your body language and facial expressions to reassure patients. By doing so, you send a message of understanding and acceptance to all patients from all backgrounds. You let patients know that you're there to help them without any bias or prejudice.

Lecturing

Your role is not to lecture patients about their health. While your job may involve educating patients about medical issues, be careful about talking too long to patients about what they should or should not do. Lecturing a patient may make him feel like a child, and it may do more harm than good. Some people rebel against lectures by doing exactly what you just told them not to do! Encourage and allow patients to take charge of their own health. Offer the patient whatever tools he needs, and then let the patient know you're available for support.

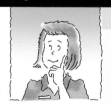

Say it Isn't So

WHEN TO USE REASSURING CLICHÉS AND LECTURES

When is it acceptable to use clichés or lectures with a patient?

A patient has just found out she has a serious health condition. She is upset and distraught. Her first comment, made in anger, is that she does not care about her life at all and would just as soon end it. Is this the time to lecture the patient about how she should be acting? Is this an appropriate time to offer a lighthearted cliché to help brighten the patient's mood?

Absolutely not! When a patient is distraught and upset, she needs support and understanding. Even if you did lecture the patient, chances are she wouldn't be listening to a word of it. Also, because of the sensitive nature of the situation, a lighthearted cliché would be out of place.

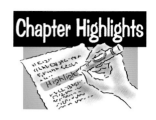

Chapter Highlights

- People have always relied on some system of communication that involves the sharing of information.
- The communication cycle includes a message and channel of communication, a receiver, a sender, and feedback.
- Communication must be complete, clear, culturally sensitive, courteous, and consistent.
- The majority of communication involves a face-to-face interaction between individuals.
- Verbal and nonverbal messages are delivered and received.
- Communication includes tone of voice, choice of words, and body posture.
- Listening skills are essential.
- Social and therapeutic communications are different and require different skill sets.
- It's important to understand the difference between social and therapeutic communication. Therapeutic communication and social communication differ in purpose and in the skills required for the communication to occur. Social communication requires nonspecific communication skills. Therapeutic communication requires specific professional, care-related skills.
- In order to be effective, the medical assistant should develop therapeutic communication skills.

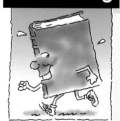

Active Learning

ACT IT OUT!

As a class, practice listening techniques. First, write down on pieces of paper several different scenarios that might occur in the medical office setting between a medical assistant and patient. Each scenario should focus on some problem or situation that the patient is facing. Fold the papers in half and put them into a box. Then, pair up with another student. Choose a scenario. One of you should play the medical assistant. The other should be the patient. Role-play the scenario two ways—showing the effective way and the ineffective way for the medical assistant to listen actively.

Chapter 3

COMMUNICATION ACROSS THE LIFESPAN

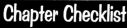

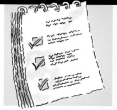

- Demonstrate an understanding of human growth and development

- Explain cognitive development theory

- List and describe Freud's three major systems or forces

- Define the reality principle and the pleasure principle

- List and describe Erikson's eight psychosocial crises

- Explain the principle of mutuality

- Define operant conditioning

- Discuss the impact of reinforcement on behavior

- Explain the significance of understanding developmental theories as they relate to approaches to communication

- Demonstrate a basic understanding of the challenges of communicating with each age group

- Describe a holistic approach to health care communication

- List communication techniques for working with children

- Describe communication techniques for working with adolescents

- Identify communication techniques for working with adults

- List and describe the therapeutic communication techniques for an older population

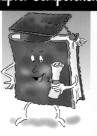

Chapter Competencies

- Adapt what is said to the recipient's level of comprehension (ABHES Competency 2.c.)
- Instruct individuals according to their needs (CAAHEP Competency 3.c.3.b.)
- Be attentive, listen, and learn (ABHES Competency 2.a.)
- Be impartial and show empathy when dealing with patients (ABHES Competency 2.b.)
- Recognize and respond to verbal and nonverbal communication (ABHES Competency 2.i., 2.k., and 2.l.; CAAHEP Competency 3.c.1.b. and 3.c.1.c.)

Language development and communication skills change throughout a person's lifespan. As a result, patients of different ages respond to and communicate about their health in different ways.

In this chapter, you'll learn about human growth and development. You'll explore the different theories of human development and behavior as described by Jean Piaget, Erik Erikson, Sigmund Freud, and B. F. Skinner. You'll also learn how these developmental theories affect your work as a health care professional and how you can communicate effectively with patients from all age groups.

Growth, Development, and Behavior and Its Impact on Communication

By learning about developmental theories, you'll discover how to communicate more effectively with each patient you encounter.

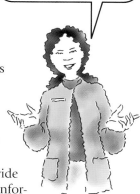

You might be wondering why it's important to learn about developmental theories and developmental stages. There are three reasons why knowing this information is helpful:

- It will affect the insights you have about what patients are experiencing.
- It will affect the way you communicate with patients at various stages of development.
- It will have an overall impact on your effectiveness as a health care professional.

Understanding development theories can also help you provide appropriate anticipatory guidance. Anticipatory guidance is information that helps a child, parent, or guardian understand what to expect as a child grows and develops. It provides information to keep children healthy as they go through different stages.

GROWTH AND DEVELOPMENT THEORIES

There are many key theories of human growth and development. No single theory is generally accepted. The theories developed by Piaget, Freud, Erikson, and Skinner have all attempted to describe how humans grow and develop through life. Understanding the basic principles of these theories will improve your communication skills as a medical assistant.

DEVELOPMENT THROUGH THE LIFESPAN

As you progress through life, you grow and develop in different ways in response to many factors. All the factors that affect your growth and development can be divided into three groups.

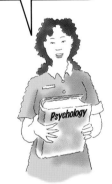

Although Freud's theories are well known, he wasn't the only psychologist to describe human growth and development! In this chapter, you'll explore several different theories that attempt to explain the stages of development.

- *Biological factors.* These are things that are passed on to you from your parents. The color of your hair and eyes, as well as your height, are some examples of biological factors.

- *Social factors.* These are factors related to your relationships, social support, environment, and culture. Your friends, religious community, and cultural traditions all have an effect on your development.

- *Psychological factors.* These factors include your self-esteem, how you cope with stress, and how you learn new information.

Piaget

In 1969, Jean Piaget, a Swiss psychologist, developed a theory of cognitive development to help explain human behavior. Piaget used his theory to describe how learning changes from infancy through adolescence.

COGNITIVE DEVELOPMENT LEARNING THEORY

Cognitive development refers to the ability to think and reason logically and to learn new ideas. Your cognitive abilities change as you grow. In simple terms, Piaget's theory states that learning is based on interaction with your environment. As a child, you gain insights, learn to solve problems, and begin to understand abstract concepts. This process can be divided into four stages.

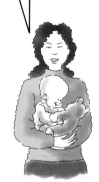

Infants use sensorimotor activities to explore new things in their environment.

1. *Sensorimotor activities.* From birth to 2 years of age, you interact with your environment using your senses and motor skills.

2. *Preoperational thought.* From 2 to 6 years of age, you interact with your environment using symbols, basic language skills, and your imagination.

3. *Concrete operational thought.* From 7 to 11 years of age, you interact with your environment using logic and reasoning, other people's perspectives, and abstract thinking.

4. *Formal operational thought.* From the age of 12 years to adulthood, you interact with your environment using a variety of hypothetical, logical, and abstract thought processes.

BASIC PRINCIPLES OF COGNITIVE DEVELOPMENT THEORY

What is cognitive development theory? There are three basic principles of Piaget's theory.

- *New experiences.* Each individual makes sense of new experiences by somehow connecting them to what is already known.

- *Sequence of development.* Every child progresses through each stage of development in the same sequence. The time frames, however, may vary from one child to the next.

- *Other influences.* Family, culture, personality, and socialization of the sexes may influence individual differences in cognitive development.

IMPORTANCE TO HEALTH CARE PROFESSIONALS

Understanding Piaget's cognitive development theory will help you communicate more effectively with patients. Use what you have learned about the different periods of cognitive development to better understand how patients of any age interact with their environment—including you!

Sigmund Freud

Austrian neurologist Sigmund Freud (1856–1939) developed a very different approach to understanding human behavior. Freud's psychoanalytic development theory emphasizes that human behavior is strongly affected by certain unconscious forces.

PSYCHOANALYTIC DEVELOPMENT THEORY

According to Freud, the basic human drives are survival and reproduction. The forces that guide these drives include hunger, thirst, avoidance of pain, and sex. But Freud pointed out that many of these forces are unconscious and hidden from a person's awareness.

MAJOR SYSTEMS OF FORCES

Freud believed that personality is made up of three basic parts:

- id
- ego
- superego

Id

The **id** is a person's basic animal nature. It includes basic drives, such as hunger and thirst, and instincts. An **instinct** is an automatic, natural behavior that does not have to be thought about. The id is mostly unconscious, selfish, pain-reducing, and pleasure-loving. It works on the **pleasure principle**—decreasing pain and increasing pleasure. Additionally, the id has very little patience. For example, if you hold a brightly colored toy in front of an infant, the infant will most likely try his hardest to grab the toy out of your hands. According to Freud, very small children are directed only by id forces. The baby does not think to ask permission for the toy. He simply grabs for what will give him the most pleasure at that time. Behavior governed mainly by the id occurs quickly and without much, if any, thought.

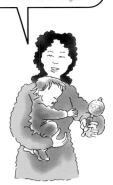

Very small children can't control their id impulses. Adults also feel driven by their id forces, but they have learned to control those urges.

Ego

The **ego** is the second of three forces behind human behavior. The ego is in touch with reality, and it develops in children between the ages of 2 and 4. The ego is aware of the world around it, and its job is to navigate around life's obstacles to satisfy the id's desires. For example, a 3-year-old child may want to play with a toy, but she also may know that if she simply grabs the toy she wants, she will be scolded. The child's ego allows her to delay gratifying her desire to have the toy until she can do so appropriately, by asking for permission. In this way, the ego works on the **reality principle**—taking care of a need as soon as an appropriate pathway or object is found.

For most adults, it's often not possible to satisfy needs and wants immediately. Sometimes, you have to tolerate pain, displeasure, or tension to gain pleasure or relief at a later time. The ego keeps track of objects, events, and people that help or hurt that process.

For example, suppose you're trying to lose weight, but you really like chocolate cake. During the first week of your diet, you had chocolate cake three times in addition to your regular meals. You managed to gain 2 pounds on your diet. At this point, your ego might begin to control those id impulses and allow you to restrain yourself from eating as much cake in the second week of your diet. In order to achieve your goal of losing weight, you may choose to have a piece of fruit instead of the cake, knowing that you may be able to have an occasional piece of chocolate cake once you achieve your goal weight.

Superego

The superego is the third of Freud's forces that drives human behavior. The **superego** represents ideal behaviors, not real behaviors. The goal of the superego is to be perfect rather than to be real or to achieve pleasure. At the center of your superego are your beliefs about what is good, bad, right, or wrong.

> The superego represents ideal behaviors, which are based on your beliefs about right and wrong.

The superego develops from the ego at about 5 years of age. As you might guess, the superego depends primarily on parents' or other caregivers' moral standards.

There are two parts of the superego:

- **conscience**—your inner understanding of punishments and warnings
- **ego ideal**—your understanding of self, formed in childhood, based on rewards and positive models

The conscience and ego ideal communicate their needs to the ego with feelings such as shame, pride, and guilt.

PSYCHOSEXUAL STAGES OF DEVELOPMENT

Freud believed that many hidden forces are tied to sexual development. He divided psychosexual development into stages. Each stage is characterized by the focus on a specific body region and the pleasure received from that particular body region.

Oral Stage

The oral stage lasts from birth to 18 months. The region of focus is the mouth. For example, an infant will explore by eating, sucking, biting, and chewing. The infant's primary need during this stage of development is security.

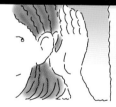

Listen to This   ID, EGO, AND SUPEREGO

Sigmund Freud thought that as humans develop, the personality moves through three main stages:

Id
- present at birth to 2 years of age
- seeks pleasure
- avoids pain
- is impatient

Ego
- develops at age 2 to 4
- delays pleasure-seeking until pleasure can be realistically achieved
- tolerates some pain if it will eventually result in pleasure
- is patient

Superego
- develops by age 5
- does what is "right" over what is pleasurable
- is motivated by fear of punishment or by internal value system
- is very patient

Anal Stage

The anal stage lasts between the ages of 18 months to 3 or 4 years. It begins when the child develops control of the anal sphincter. Children in this stage of development learn to control their bowel functions during toilet training.

Phallic Stage

Children experiencing this stage of development may be anywhere from 3 to 5, 6, or 7 years old. The region of focus is the genital area, and children often have an increased interest in gender differences. Curiosity about the genital area and masturbation are common during this stage.

Latency Stage

The latency stage marks the child's transition to the genital stage during adolescence. It occurs between the ages of 5, 6, or 7 years and puberty (which usually occurs at about 12 years). Freud thought that the sexual impulse is repressed during this stage in the service of learning. During the latency stage, children identify with the parent of the same sex in preparing for adult roles and relationships.

Genital Stage

The genital stage begins at puberty and lasts through adulthood. It begins with the reappearance of the adolescent's sex drive. Teenagers often focus on the pleasure of sexual intercourse during this stage. As they make adjustments in relationships, teens may have difficulty dealing with sexual pressures and conflicts. During this final stage of psychosexual development, a person develops a strong sexual interest in the opposite sex. Freud thought that to achieve this stage, you need to have a balance of work and love.

IMPORTANCE TO HEALTH CARE PROFESSIONALS

In the mentally healthy person, the id, ego, and superego must work together to allow the person to fulfill basic needs and desires. When these three forces are at odds, a person will show signs of *maladjustment* (being poorly adjusted). By understanding how these three forces affect behavior, you as a medical assistant can more easily determine patients' abilities to meet their own basic needs.

Erik Erikson

Born in Germany, psychologist Erik Erikson (1902–1994) became an American citizen and focused on child psychoanalysis. Remember that Freud described human behavior based on psychosexual development. In contrast, Erikson felt there was a strong connection between society and the way personality develops. As a result, Erikson described behavior based on psychosocial factors.

PSYCHOSOCIAL CRISES

Erikson accepted Freud's theories but with an important difference—he thought that the effects of society and culture on personality are critical to development. Erikson's psychosocial theory is based on his belief that the stages of development include psychosocial **crises** that must be mastered.

One example of a crisis is *trust versus mistrust,* which occurs during infancy. Erikson believed that we must learn balance. As infants, we need to learn mostly trust; but we also need to learn a little mistrust, so as not to grow up to become gullible. During each stage of development, the child or adult tries to resolve the crisis and is either successful or unsuccessful.

THE EPIGENETIC PRINCIPLE

Erikson used the epigenetic principle to form his psychosocial theory of development. The **epigenetic principle** states that development happens as personality unfolds in a preset plan. And this plan, according to Erikson, is made up of eight stages. Characteristics of each stage include the following:

- *Crises or tasks.* Crises characterize each stage of development. Being able to move through each stage depends on your success or failure at resolving previous crises.

- *Virtues.* If you succeed at a certain crisis, you take on a psychosocial strength. This strength helps you through the remaining stages of development.

- *Malignancies and maladaptations.* Not moving well through a stage results in malignancies and maladaptations. These endanger future develop-ment. A *malignancy* develops when there is too little of the positive and too much of the nega-tive aspect of a crisis or task. An example might be a person who can't trust others. A *maladapta-tion* develops when there is too much of the positive and too little of the negative aspect of a certain task. An example might be a person who trusts others too much.

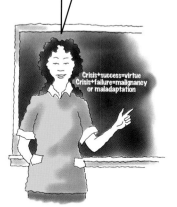

The crises or tasks at each stage of development may result in the development of virtues or malignancies and maladaptations.

ERIKSON'S EIGHT STAGES

According to Erikson's psychosocial theory, people move through eight stages as they progress from birth to death. Each of these stages has some crisis, or task, connected to it. You might master this crisis or you might not. But your success or failure with the crisis affects what happens as you progress through the remaining stages. Also, each stage lasts only a certain time period and takes place at a certain pace.

The next sections describe Erikson's eight stages of psycho-social development in order as they occur from birth to old age.

Trust Versus Mistrust

The first stage occurs during infancy, or during the first year or year and a half of life. Infants must develop trust without completely eliminating the ability to mistrust. If an infant's parents or caregivers meet his basic needs (such as warmth, food, and comfort), the child will develop the feeling that the world is a safe place. He sees people as generally reliable and loving. However, if the infant's parents or caregivers provide unreliable or inadequate care, the child will be apprehensive and suspicious around people. And if parents provide too much comfort or shelter from the outside world, the child may learn to be too trusting of others.

Autonomy Versus Shame and Doubt

From the age of about 18 months to 3 or 4 years, toddlers seek a degree of **autonomy,** or independence, while minimizing shame and doubt. If children are permitted to explore and manipulate their environment at this stage, they will develop a sense of autonomy as well as a level of self-control and self-esteem. For example, when a child comes to a physician's practice, you may offer the child the choice of having her height taken first or being weighed first. This helps to give the child a sense of control and can foster independence by allowing her to make a decision.

If a child is unable to explore and assert independence, she may develop a sense of shame and doubt. She may give up and stop trying to be autonomous, or she may develop compulsive behaviors to compensate for her lack of confidence. If the child does not learn any shame and doubt, though, she may become impulsive in her actions, rather than learning to control her behaviors.

Initiative Versus Guilt

During the preschool years, or when children are between the ages of three and six years old, they must learn to develop initiative. This task can be hindered if a child experiences too much guilt during this stage in development.

Initiative is a positive response to challenges. When a child develops initiative, she assumes responsibilities, learns new skills, and feels purposeful. At this stage, children learn to take initiative in learning by seeking new experiences and exploring the "how" and "why" of activities. It's the response a

Send and Receive

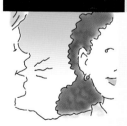

AUTONOMY TALK

Suppose that you must treat a 3-year-old patient. The child is naturally curious about the instruments and other objects in the examination room. What is the best way to communicate to the child that many of these things are not for play? How can you use what you know about developmental stages to effectively communicate with the child? What is the best way to preserve the child's autonomy and still maintain the child's safety? Here are some examples of ineffective and effective dialogue to use in this situation.

Ineffective:

- Zachary is a 3-year-old boy who is not feeling well. His mother has brought him in to be examined by the physician. You meet with Zachary first to take his vital signs.

- "Hi, Zachary! I hear you're not feeling so well today. Well, let's have you sit in this chair over here while I examine you. Now, do not touch anything in here, okay? Just sit and be patient."

- Seconds later, Zachary reaches for one of the instruments on the counter. "Zachary, put that down." Zachary becomes frustrated and picks up a different instrument hanging on the wall. "No, Zachary, put that down!" Zachary becomes agitated, pouting.

- Minutes later, the effectiveness of your interaction with Zachary is low. Zachary's sense of shame and frustration is rising.

Children at this stage are naturally curious. They want to explore by holding and touching. Creating a safe environment for children in this stage is critically important. Allowing the child to explore safely is key.

Effective:

- "Hi, Zachary! I hear you're not feeling so well. Look what I have for you!" Show Zachary a box of age-appropriate toys for him to play with while you take his vital signs.

- "These are for you to play with while I examine you. Okay?" Zachary is happy. He is able to satisfy his curiosity and preserve his autonomy safely. You can proceed with your examination without distraction.

An examination room can be a scary place for many children at this or any stage of development. It can be scary for adults, too! Providing fun but safe activities to ease a child's fears helps the examination progress more smoothly. More importantly, it helps preserve the child's sense of autonomy.

child receives to these activities that determines whether her sense of initiative remains intact. If a child is encouraged to seek new experiences and to learn, she will be more likely to attempt more challenging language and motor skills. But if the child is restricted from learning new things, she will feel a sense of guilt for her actions.

> Preschool-aged children are curious about their environment and may ask many questions to find out the "how" and "why" of activities.

Industry Versus Inferiority

School-aged children (6 to 12 years old) begin to focus on the end result of tasks and to seek recognition for their accomplishments. For example, a child may paint a picture to receive praise from a parent or teacher. To progress through this stage successfully, children must develop a capacity for industry while avoiding a sense of inferiority.

During this stage, a child's social circle broadens to include teachers and peers. Along with the new knowledge gained in school, the child also learn basic social skills. Ideally, the child develops a sense of competency by completing tasks and receiving praise or recognition for these tasks. The praise can take place in social areas, academics, or athletics. If the child is rejected during this stage and feels unsuccessful, he will develop a sense of inferiority or incompetence.

Identity Versus Role Confusion

From the start of puberty to the age of about 18 or 20 years, individuals develop a sense of self. During this stage of development, the key is to achieve ego identity while avoiding role confusion.

To achieve **ego identity** means to know who you are and how you fit in with the rest of society. A person who has successfully mastered this crisis has taken all she has learned about life and herself and molded it into a unified meaningful self-image. Without ego identity, however, the person will have role confusion—uncertainty about her place in society and the world. When role confusion occurs, an identity crisis results.

Intimacy Versus Isolation

This stage of development occurs during young adulthood, or between the ages of 18 and about 30 years. However, the age at which this stage occurs varies dramatically from person to person. During this stage, individuals must achieve some degree of intimacy to avoid isolation.

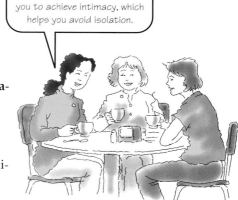

Having close friends allows you to achieve intimacy, which helps you avoid isolation.

Intimacy is the ability to be close to others and to participate in society. **Isolation** is the removal of one's self from love, friendship, and community. By developing relationships and making commitments to other people, you achieve intimacy. The fear of making intimate connections creates isolation and loneliness.

Generativity Versus Stagnation

During middle adulthood, or somewhere between the mid-20s and late 50s, people attempt to achieve the proper balance between generativity and stagnation.

Generativity is a concern for the next generation and all future generations. **Stagnation** is being self-absorbed and obsessed with your own needs. This is the stage of the "midlife crisis." Sometimes, you may take a look at your life and ask, "What am I doing with my life?" When you feel that you're making a contribution to the world, you'll have a capacity for caring that will serve you through the rest of your life.

Ego Integrity Versus Despair

In late adulthood—somewhere around 60 years of age—individuals must develop ego integrity with a minimal amount of despair.

Ego integrity is the ability to reflect on the course of your life, including the choices you have made, and to come to terms with your life as you have lived it. With ego integrity comes

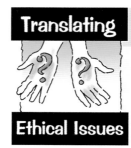

Translating Ethical Issues

HELPING PATIENTS COPE WITH DESPAIR

Here are some ethical tips to remember when interacting with patients in the ego integrity versus despair stage of development.

- Remember to listen attentively to a patient who may need to express her feelings of despair. Keeping this information confidential is critically important.

- Remind the patient of available resources, such as family, friends, spirituality, or counseling, to help her cope with feelings of despair.

- Document any concerns you have regarding a patient's feelings of despair. If the patient is openly suicidal, or if you have reason to believe the patient could be suicidal, notify the physician immediately.

wisdom. Despair develops if you become preoccupied with the past, your failures, or your regrets.

THE PRINCIPLE OF MUTUALITY

All of Erikson's stages of development are united by the principle of **mutuality**. This principle refers to the interaction of generations.

Although many theorists believe that parents influence their children's development, Erikson believed that children influence their parents' development as well. For example, parents experience certain life changes when they have children. Erikson's principle of mutuality states that the lives of parents and children are interconnected. In Erikson's own words, "Healthy children will not fear life if their elders have integrity enough not to fear death." This quote illustrates how an elder adult's success during the ego integrity versus despair stage can have a lasting impact on a child moving through the other stages of development.

This principle gives us a framework to talk about how our culture compares to other cultures. It also allows us to reflect on life as it is today as compared with a few centuries ago. Erikson and other researchers have found that the general pattern of interconnectedness across generations has held true over many centuries and across all cultures.

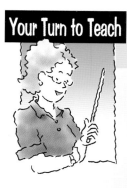

PATIENT EDUCATION: CHILD DEVELOPMENT STAGES

Psychologist Erik Erikson described eight stages of development from birth to old age. During each stage, a particular developmental task should be accomplished. By educating patients about these eight stages, you help increase patient awareness and knowledge. Patients can use the information presented in the table to understand themselves as well as those with whom they interact.

Erikson's Psychosocial Theory of Development	
Developmental Crisis/Task	**Stage**
Trust versus mistrust	infancy
Autonomy versus shame and doubt	toddler
Initiative versus guilt	preschool
Industry versus inferiority	school age
Identity versus role confusion	adolescence
Intimacy versus isolation	young adulthood
Generativity versus stagnation	middle adulthood
Ego integrity versus despair	later adulthood

B. F. Skinner

B. F. Skinner was an American pioneer in the field of psychology during the 1900s. He became well known for his study of behavioral learning theories.

BEHAVIORAL LEARNING THEORIES

Many behavioral learning theories explore the relationship between a stimulus and a response. Skinner based his work on the work of an earlier researcher named Ivan Pavlov. By studying animals' responses to various stimuli, Pavlov developed theories we now know as *classical conditioning* and the *conditioned response*. Pavlov's most famous experiment involved dogs and their responses to the stimulus of food. Every time Pavlov brought food to the dogs, he rang a bell. Over time, the dogs learned to associate the bell-ringing with receiving food. Any time Pavlov rang the bell, the dogs would begin to drool, whether they smelled food or not. The dogs became *conditioned* to associate bell-ringing with food, and their bodies reacted just as if food were actually present.

Skinner took these theories one step further. He based his experiments on the principle that rewarded behavior will be repeated, and, conversely, that unrewarded behavior will not be repeated.

OPERANT CONDITIONING

The heart of Skinner's work focused on **operant condition-ing**. According to Skinner, you "operate" in your environment by doing what you do. In the process of "operating," you come upon many different stimuli. A stimulus may reinforce a behav-ior that you do, or it may cause you to stop a behavior you had been doing.

Here are some basic principles associated with operant conditioning:

- Operant conditioning occurs when the "operant" performs a certain behavior before reinforcement is given.

- Every behavior is followed by a consequence. The nature of the consequence determines whether the behavior will occur again in the future.

- Reinforcement is a type of consequence that increases the chance of a behavior happening again. With **continu-ous reinforcement**, every time a behavior happens, it's reinforced. However, with **intermittent reinforcement**, a behavior is reinforced only at certain intervals.

Let's use an example to understand how operant condition-ing works. Suppose you're about to meet a new patient for the first time. You walk into the examination room and immedi-ately greet the new patient with a friendly smile and a warm hello. Likewise, the patient responds by smiling and saying hello.

Whenever you greet another person, the other person responds in some way. Your greeting is a behavior; the other person's response is the consequence. In the example, your behavior (your greeting) produces a positive response (the patient's smile and warm hello.)

If patients always responded warmly to your greeting, this would be a continuous reinforcement of your behavior. But, realistically, some patients may not respond warmly to your greeting—this would be an intermittent reinforcement of your behavior. Since you enjoy receiving a warm response back from your patients, you'll most likely continue to greet each patient warmly. Operant conditioning has trained you to greet patients in a warm and friendly manner.

> If every patient you greet responds with a smile and a friendly greeting of his own, this continuous reinforcement will encourage you to keep greeting patients in a pleasant manner.

WHY OPERANT CONDITIONING MATTERS TO YOU

You're shaped by your environment to enjoy certain things that you do well. When you receive positive reinforcement for something you do, you want to repeat the action.

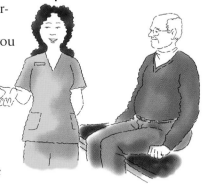

It's important to understand the significance of reinforcement and its effect on behavior. By doing so, you'll be better equipped to recognize and understand certain patterns of behavior in yourself and in the patients you encounter. By understanding how operant conditioning works, you'll be able to communicate with patients more effectively regarding health care issues.

Different Age Groups Communicate Differently

You do not need to be a psychologist to notice that people of different age groups communicate differently.

For example, a 7-year-old boy with an infected wound is probably not interested in understanding the process that led to his infection. He knows one thing—he wants his painful cut to feel better. Taking time to explain how infection happens would

Summary of Some Human Growth and Development Theories			
Piaget	**Freud**	**Erikson**	**Skinner**
Cognitive Development Theory: Stages include sensorimotor activities, preoperational thought, concrete operational thought, and formal operational thought.	*Psychoanalytic Development Theory:* Three basic parts of personality are identified as the id, ego, and superego. *Psychosexual Development Theory:* Stages include oral, anal, phallic, latency, and genital.	*Psychosocial Development Theory:* Eight stages of growth from infancy to later adulthood and development crises or tasks at each (e.g., trust versus mistrust during infancy) are identified.	*Behavioral Learning Theory of Operant Conditioning:* The nature of a consequence to a behavior determines whether the behavior will occur again.

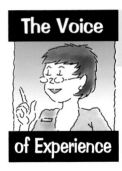

The Voice of Experience

OPERANT CONDITIONING AND PATIENT CARE

Q: *I am currently working with a patient who has stopped taking her ulcer medication. She claims that when she took it last, it didn't help and her ulcer was just as painful. How can I help this patient understand that the ulcer medication will help when taken properly?*

A: It's possible that the patient took the medication at the wrong time. For certain ulcer medications to work effectively, the patient must take the medication before meals, not after. If the patient takes the medication too late, she will still experience pain from her ulcer after a meal, and this will cause her to be less likely to take it again in the future.

This is an opportunity to use operant conditioning to train the patient to use her medication effectively. Here's what is happening:

1. First, the patient has a meal (the behavior).
2. Next, the patient experiences pain after the meal (the consequence).

To use operant conditioning to improve this situation, tell the patient that the medication must be taken before eating. This way, the pain (a negative consequence) is eliminated. Instead, the patient experiences no pain (a positive consequence). Once the patient experiences a pain-free meal by taking the ulcer medication at the right time, she will be more inclined to continue taking her medication regularly.

be useless in this case. The boy would be bored before you could say "white blood cells"!

On the other hand, a 50-year-old man with a similar wound might *want* you to explain how his wound got infected. He has the ability to understand the process. He *wants* to understand the process. The knowledge helps him take responsibility for his own healing.

GROWTH AND DEVELOPMENT

As you grow and develop, your self-concept, self-image, and self-confidence change. As a result, the way you communicate with others changes, too. Before you can have effective therapeutic communication with patients, think about how you would want to be approached now as opposed to how you would have wanted to be approached 10, 15, or 20 years ago. This is a good starting point for understanding how others respond to your communication technique.

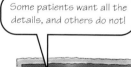

Some patients want all the details, and others do not!

Understanding the stages of growth and development will help you communicate effectively with patients as well as with their family members and support team. Learning how to respond appropriately with the right communication tools and skills will strengthen all of your patient interactions.

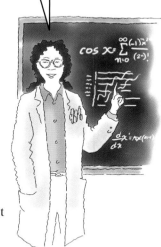

HOLISTIC APPROACH

One of the most valuable tips to remember in your interactions with patients is this: treat the whole patient, not just the condition. This approach to patient care is called a **holistic** approach. When you first meet a patient, consider the patient's gender, culture, age, occupation, environment, genetics, and life experiences. Take all these things into consideration. They are part of who your patient is. Let them guide you in the way you approach the patient's health care.

For example, you may assist one patient who is an older adult male who speaks English as a second language, comes from a large family, and teaches nuclear physics. You may then assist an adolescent female patient who speaks no English, is an only child, and attends middle school. These two patients require completely different communication approaches. You use different words, gestures, and expressions to send your messages to each patient.

The holistic approach to health care means that you consider everything about the patient. Using a holistic approach, you can help each patient get the best medical care possible.

AGE ISN'T JUST A NUMBER!

A patient's age has a big effect on the way you can best help her. You must learn how to communicate with patients of all ages. In this chapter, you'll learn specific communication skills to use with four different age groups:

- children
- adolescents
- adults
- older adults

With small children, for example, it's especially important to address safety issues. Also remember that children become fearful easily. Sharing too much medical information with very young patients might frighten them. Instruct a child in a way that will help him stay safe without becoming afraid. This is important in your communications with this young age group.

Older children and adolescents might be seeing a physician only because their parent insisted they do so. Communicating with a patient who never wanted to see the physician in the first place can be tricky.

Adults offer a different challenge. Many adults have to juggle their personal, social, and work activities. Family, school, work, social, and religious interests all affect the way an adult patient approaches his own health care. An adult patient may know he needs to see a physician, but he may be stressed about having to spend time in a physician's office. This, in turn, affects communications between you and the adult patient.

Older adults offer yet another challenge. Some older adult patients have problems with memory loss and confusion or suffer from overall poor health. On the other hand, other older adult patients may be quite curious about their health and eager to learn as much as they can.

One of your goals as a medical assistant is to understand the challenges of each age group and of each individual within an age group. Accomplishing this goal plays a big part in your ability to communicate with all patients.

COMMUNICATION TECHNIQUES

When you communicate with patients from different age groups, you'll need to change your technique to match the age group of the patient. There are four general rules you can keep in mind to help increase the effectiveness of your communications with all patients.

1. Always speak directly, and give the patient your full attention.

2. Always speak clearly. Make sure your messages are clearly stated and easy to understand.

3. Always check for the patient's understanding. Ask the patient if he has any questions, and make sure the patient understands what is being said to him.

4. Always pay attention to the verbal and nonverbal messages the patient is sending you. Ask for clarification if you're unsure of what the patient is trying to say.

5. Ask patients to repeat instructions or to demonstrate what you have taught. Write down instructions for patients and/or their caregiver(s).

One specific communication technique you can use is choosing the right words for the right patient. Choosing age-appropriate words when communicating with patients is a critical part of what you do. The way you instruct a child about how to care for a bandaged wound is different from the way you instruct an adult. With a child, you might use a stuffed animal to demonstrate how to keep a bandaged area clean and dry. But with an adult, using a stuffed animal would be perceived as condescending. This chapter will discuss techniques you can use to communicate effectively with each age group.

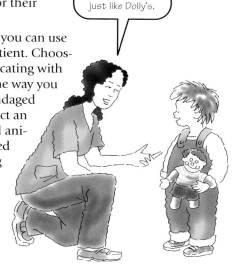

Chatting with Children

The branch of medicine that deals with children is called **pediatric** medicine. Children have specific health issues that a pediatric physician specializes in. Children also have specific communication needs that you, as a medical assistant, must learn how to address.

CHILDREN WITH ILLNESSES

Individual children respond to illness differently. Some may seem quiet and withdrawn. Others may be unable to sit still for more than a few seconds. Some children may revert to certain comfort behaviors, like sucking their thumbs or cuddling a favorite blanket or toy. Many children are fearful of seeing a physician. Some children might think being ill or getting hurt is a punishment.

In any case, all children who are ill or hurt share one thing—they want to feel better. Learning how to address each child's individual differences *and* respond to the child's illness are two of your biggest challenges.

EFFECTIVE COMMUNICATIONS WITH KIDS

The approach you take when speaking to children is critical. Your words, tone, and body language may be slightly different for each child. You must learn to change your communication

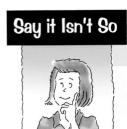

Say it Isn't So

COMMUNICATING WITH CHILDREN WHO ARE ILL

How do I talk to a four-year-old about his illness?

Suppose you're treating a 4-year-old for an illness. You can plainly see that the child is scared and does not understand why she is feeling ill. Should you explain in detail to the child how the illness started, its symptoms, its pathological nature, and all possible treatments and outcomes?

Of course not! At 4 years of age, children are able to use only basic language skills. Speak to the child in simple terms. For example, if you notice the child leaning forward or crying, you could ask "It looks like you're crying. Does your tummy hurt? Can you point to where it hurts?" If possible, keep words to one or two syllables. Reassure the child using easy-to-understand words and a gentle voice.

style to suit the needs of each child you see. Here are some guidelines:

1. Talk at eye level. Either come down to the child's level, or bring the child up to yours. It's important that you're on the same eye-to-eye level when communicating with children.

2. Speak gently. A child who is already scared about a visit with a physician responds better to a gentle tone. Use your voice to soothe and calm, rather than to excite and agitate.

3. Move slowly and visibly. Children are excellent observers! Make sure all your movements are slow and easily seen.

4. Announce your touch. Always tell a child when you need to touch him. You do not want to startle the child by suddenly taking his arm for a blood pressure reading.

5. Say it again. Rephrase questions or comments if the child does not understand. Ask the child if he understands what you just said.

6. Toy talk. Use a stuffed animal to help break the communication barrier with a child. Ask how Teddy is feeling first. Put a bandage on Teddy to demonstrate what you're about to do to the child.

7. Crying is okay. Allow a child to cry. Ask if Teddy is crying, too!

Form a Relationship

Many children have the same feelings as adult patients. They are scared, and they need help. But children are still growing and developing as human beings. So the behaviors connected to a child's feelings are different from those of an adult. A child who is scared might "act out" her fear by throwing things, yelling, or hitting. For this reason, it may be harder to form a relationship with a child than with an adult.

Here's a tip for your first interaction with a child: use something to break the ice. Remember to make eye contact and to speak directly to the child. Let the child know you're there to help, not to hurt. Perhaps offering a colorful book or magazine, a box of crayons and a coloring book, or a stuffed toy will do the trick. Start out your interaction with a child on the right foot. By doing so, you help guarantee a successful visit for everybody.

Environment

As with all patients, make sure the examination room for children is quiet and private. Provide some safe activities to help keep the child busy. If the waiting period gets too long, check back often to make sure the child (and whoever is with the child) is okay.

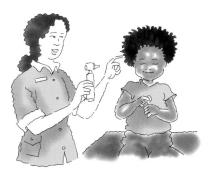

It might be helpful to explain some of the medical equipment in the room. For example, use simple words and terms to tell the child what a stethoscope, otoscope, or sphygmomanometer do.

Find ways to make children feel more comfortable.

Listen

Remember that more than half of good communication involves listening. When you interact with children, take time to listen carefully and politely to what they have to say. If you ask a question, wait for the child to answer completely. Do not interrupt. Some children may take a while to answer a question completely. Be patient and sensitive to a child's need for extra time. Watch for nonverbal clues, such as clutching a sore part of the body, which can tell you more about what the child is trying to say.

Also, be sure to listen to any questions or concerns the parent or caregiver might have. If a child must be held still, ask the adult if she would prefer to hold the child. The child might be more comfortable having a familiar person hold him.

Choice

Let children "help" during an examination. Give children choices whenever possible. Ask a child if she wants to hold the roll of bandages or the adhesive tape while you dress a wound. Ask a child if she would like to have her temperature or blood pressure taken first. Ask if she would like her caregiver or you to hold her during an examination.

Giving children choices during an examination or procedure makes them feel more in control of the situation. This allows them to feel like they are taking a bigger part in their health care.

Talking with Teens

Adolescence is characterized as a period full of rapid growth and development. Some literature suggests that adolescence is the stage of life from ages 10 to 20. Other literature suggests that adolescence is from ages 12 to 18. However, experts agree that adolescence does not have a distinct beginning or end.

For patients in this age group, the body is going through many physical changes. An adolescent patient's peers (people in her own age group) play a major role in her life, and self-concept is starting to stabilize. The need for independence is strong in adolescents. Body image is a high priority.

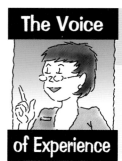

The Voice of Experience

WORKING WITH CHILDREN WHO ARE FEARFUL OF INJECTIONS

Q: *What can I do when very young patients are so scared of getting an injection that they scream and cling to their parent?*

A: Once a child is already crying before an injection, it may be difficult to calm him down. Above all, stay calm yourself! Children sense your own fear and tension. Staying calm and gentle will help keep a child from becoming more fearful. One handy tip to use with children who are able to talk is to tell them to take a deep breath and blow out during the injection. Using a party noisemaker to blow out can help a child cope with this procedure. Tell the child that he can make as much noise as he wants when he blows into the noisemaker during the injection. This activity may help take his focus off the injection, so the child will not be as acutely aware of the pain.

An adolescent's attitude toward adults may be negative or positive. Some adolescents may resent authority figures. You may meet an adolescent patient for the first time and find that you're unable to keep consistent eye contact with her. The patient may refuse to look at you at all. She may not speak to you, either. Or the adolescent patient may want to say something to you, but may feel uncomfortable or silly doing so.

Your interactions with adolescent patients present many unique challenges. Understanding or remembering how it must feel to be going through so many changes at this time will help you interact more effectively.

THOSE TRICKY TEENAGE YEARS

It's tough being a teenager. The body is changing; feelings are changing; goals are changing. Adulthood is approaching fast; life is scary and exciting all at the same time. Sexual characteristics develop. Boys develop facial hair and a lower voice, and they begin to produce sperm. Girls develop breasts and body hair, and they experience their first menstruation. Along with these changes comes a spurt in general physical growth. For most teenagers, full adult size is reached during adolescence. With all of these physical changes, it's easy to see why body image is so important during this stage.

With developing sexual characteristics comes the ability to reproduce. Adolescents may have different levels of understanding about reproduction and sexual relations. Some adolescents may be sexually active; others may not. Some adolescents may have a close relationship with one or both of their parents; others may not. These are some of the issues you should be aware of when interacting with adolescent patients.

EFFECTIVE ADOLESCENT CHITCHAT

Communicating with adolescents can be tricky. But it can also be wonderful. Always remember that all patients, including adolescents, want to feel better. Your job is to give patients the tools and information they need to feel healthy. Adolescents may not know why they are feeling ill. They may not understand how to keep themselves healthy. Also, they may not understand critical health information. As a medical assistant, there may be times when you need to educate an adolescent patient about diet and exercise. Using visual aids such as posters or diagrams may help. You may also direct an adolescent patient to a specific website. Have posters, pamphlets, videos, or other aids handy if and when the opportunity to use them arises.

Privacy

Adolescents are a special case under the HIPAA privacy regulation. This regulation generally defers to state law on the issue of parents and minors. The American Medical Association encourages physicians to involve parents in the care of their adolescent children unless it interferes with the patient's health care.

Some adolescents may be uncomfortable sharing personal information with their parent or caregiver in the room. Some may want to share personal information only with the physician. Be sure to ask the patient what his preference is. If necessary, kindly ask parents or caregivers to leave the examination room for a few minutes.

Choice

Always give the adolescent patient an opportunity to make choices about his health treatment. This is part of learning how to be a responsible adult. It might be easier for some adoles-

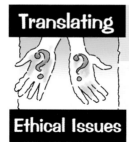

Translating

Ethical Issues

ADOLESCENT PATIENTS AND CONFIDENTIALITY RIGHTS

It's important for you to know how to best approach the issue of confidentiality in adolescent health care. Here are some tips to keep in mind:

- Always respond to the needs of all adolescent patients. Let them know you'll help them in any way possible.

- Regarding their health care, encourage adolescents to involve their parents or caregivers. Although it may not always be possible, it's important for adolescents to be able to work together with their parents or caregivers.

- Explain to both the adolescent and her parents or caregivers that the adolescent has the right to private examination and counseling.

- In some cases, the physician might need to share certain information with a parent or caregiver. Information that affects the well-being of the patient or of somebody else falls into this category. Explain to the adolescent under what circumstances information will be shared with a parent or caregiver.

cents to make health care choices when a parent or caregiver is not present. Be sure to look for nonverbal clues that might indicate this.

For example, you might ask an adolescent a question that appears to make him uncomfortable. He may look nervously to his parent before trying to respond. You may want to ask the adolescent if there is something he would like to discuss in private. If he responds positively, politely ask the parent to step outside for a few minutes. With the parent out of the examination room, ask the adolescent if he would like to answer the questions or discuss them with the physician.

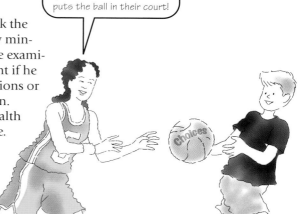

Allowing adolescent patients to make choices puts the ball in their court!

Give adolescent patients health care choices whenever possible. Explain privacy options, treatment options, medication options, and appointment options. Letting the patient choose puts the ball in his court.

Dignity and Respect

A key to communicating with adolescents is staying open, honest, and respectful. Help adolescents maintain their **dignity**, or feeling of being worthy. **Respect** them. That is, show your admiration for their qualities, abilities, or achievements. Avoid sending messages that blame, put down, or belittle. Your goal is to make the adolescent patient feel better about herself, not worse. Be supportive, not judgmental.

"I" Messages

A critical skill in communicating with adolescent patients is learning to use "I" messages instead of "you" messages. Many adolescents are very sensitive and can perceive casual statements as judgmental messages. Learning to communicate in a way that shows respect to an adolescent is a valuable skill to master.

For example, suppose you're seeing an adolescent patient who is complaining about stomach cramps. The patient keeps avoiding answering your questions. Here are two ways you could respond to the patient:

- *Ineffective.* "You keep avoiding my questions. Why are you doing that?"

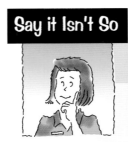

Say it Isn't So

DO PARENTS HAVE THE RIGHT TO BE INFORMED ABOUT AN ADOLESCENT'S MEDICAL CONDITION?

What if an adolescent does not want to be examined with his parent present, but his parent refuses to leave the examination room?

A 15-year-old boy and his mother come to the office. The boy has shoulder pain. During your interview with the boy, he asks that his mother not be in the room when the physician examines him. You ask the mother to leave the room, but she says that she has a right to be present. Should you allow her to stay?

It's important to understand that patients have the right to be examined in a private setting. Many adolescents may be more comfortable being examined without their parents present. However, parents do have the right to be informed about the health of their minor children. In this case, you should quietly and calmly explain to the mother that her son has asked to be examined without her in the room. Be sure to add that the physician will share with her any information related to her son's health.

- *Effective.* "I'm getting the feeling these questions make you uncomfortable. Is there anything I can do to make it easier for you to answer them?"

Communicating with an adolescent patient using "I" messages keeps blame and judgmental statements out of the conversation. It also gives the patient the opportunity to take a more active part in her communications with you.

Honesty

Without honesty in a patient interaction, the quality of your communication is decreased. You may find that adolescents are especially sensitive to your honesty or lack thereof. Patients of all age groups should feel they can trust you. They should know that you're there to help them with all of their health care needs.

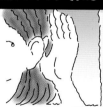

Listen to This | "I" MESSAGES

The chart below contains some ways to turn messages into "I" messages. The column on the left contains some "You" messages that place blame or are judgmental. The column on the right contains the same message turned into an "I" message.

Turning "You" Messages into "I" Messages

"You" Message	"I" Message
"You need to control your anger."	"I see that you're angry right now."
"You're avoiding my questions."	"I feel like I might be using the wrong words to ask my questions."
	"I feel like my questions are making you uncomfortable."
"You need to take better care of yourself."	"I see that you're not feeling well."

Communicating with Adults

Adults have many more experiences with health-related situations than either adolescents or children. Some of these experiences may have been positive, while others may have been negative. Also, the health-related information that adults have might be incorrect. For example, some adults may have been told by their parents or grandparents that when they are sick, they should eat more. But often when you're not feeling well, eating food, especially heavy food, produces nausea and even vomiting. This can slow down the healing process.

Communicating with adults requires that you consider their many life experiences. Be aware of the ways in which these experiences influence the adult's attitude about health. Also look for clues about any incorrect health information adult patients may have.

ADULTHOOD

The lifestyle of the adult patient is very different from that of the adolescent. Most adults spend every day trying to balance their careers, personal relationships, and family commitments. And most adults have been doing this for years. Some adults have more obligations to balance than others do. Some adults are simply better at balancing life's pressures than others are.

The most important thing to keep in mind when dealing with adult patients is that the responsibility of caring for themselves, their partners, their children, and, in some cases, their own parents, can be quite stressful. This constant stress is often a major factor affecting the health of adult patients.

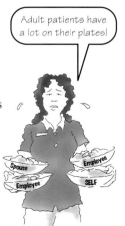

Adult patients have a lot on their plates!

TECHNIQUES FOR THERAPEUTIC COMMUNICATION WITH ADULTS

Keep in mind the lifestyle of your adult patients. This is the first step in being able to respond to and communicate with them effectively. Here are some more ways that you can strengthen your interactions with adult patients.

Individual Information

With adult patients, you must develop a sense of how much information the patient wants to know. One patient might want to know every detail about his condition. Another patient might prefer not knowing the details.

Remember that the adult patient has most likely been living in a set routine for many years. Most adult patients know themselves well. They know what works for them and what does not. They know what their needs are regarding information, relationships, interactions, and communication. Respect these needs when you interact with adult patients. And if you sense the patient isn't sure what he needs to know regarding a medical diagnosis, begin by repeating the essential information originally given by the physician. Then branch out with some questions for the patient, such as, "This medication needs to be taken under specific conditions that are listed on the bottle. Do you want me to go over these conditions with you here at the office?"

Delivery

The way you deliver messages to the patient has a major effect on how well your interaction with the patient will go. Make sure your messages are clear. Choose words that you know the patient will easily understand, without treating the patient like a child. Ask for feedback to determine if the patient understands what you have told him.

For example, suppose you have to do a throat culture to see if a patient has strep throat. First, you must swab the patient's throat for the culture. Most adult patients would think it rude if you were to abruptly walk into the examination room, swab in hand, tell the patient to open his mouth, and then take the culture. They would expect you to first greet them, then explain the procedure you're about to perform, and then give them a moment to ask questions or relax and ready themselves for the procedure.

Explanations

Provide explanations that the patient can remember and understand. Here are some tips for positive explanations:

- Using complex medical terms is generally not an effective way to communicate with patients. Most patients are not familiar with such terms and prefer simpler words.

- Because many adults lead very busy lives, it might be helpful to write down all important information related to a treatment. Provide information sheets or pamphlets if they are available.

- Verify that the patient has understood your message by asking questions and listening to the patient's response.

Make your communication with adults as interactive as possible. Encourage patients to provide feedback so you know if your message is being interpreted correctly.

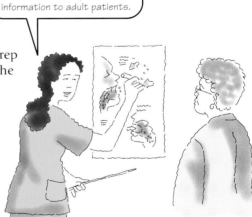

Take the time to explain medical information to adult patients.

Let's say the patient's throat culture has come back positive for strep throat. The physician has informed the patient of the results, but you sense that the patient is still not sure what this means. Ask the patient if he has any questions, and do your best to answer them—always keeping your scope of practice in mind. If you're unsure whether you should be answering a question, it may be better instead to pass the question on to the physician.

Planning and Collaboration

For the adult patient, any treatment plan means an addition to her already busy life. So it's important for you to sit down with the adult patient to make sure she understands and can follow the treatment plan as prescribed. For example, help the patient figure out the best way to remember to take medication. Involving the patient in her own treatment plan strengthens the patient's sense of responsibility. It also helps guarantee that the patient will follow the treatment and get well.

Relationships

From your first interaction with any patient, one of your goals is to build a lasting and effective relationship. Finding ways to connect positively with every patient only helps strengthen your interactions and ability to communicate effectively. Here are some questions you can ask yourself to help you start your patient relationships on the right foot.

- *What support does the patient need?* With adult patients, try to provide whatever support is necessary to help them balance their full schedules with any treatment plan they must follow. Encourage adult patients to call with any questions or concerns they might have. If possible, call them to see if they are having any problems following their treatment plan.

- *What is your objective?* Know what your objective is with each patient. Keep your objective clear. This will help you communicate more clearly with the patient. Your objective might only be to take blood pressure and temperature. Or your objective might be to explain how to take a particular medication. Clarifying your objective helps both you and the patient.

- *What kind of environment does the patient need?* Be aware of the physical and emotional needs of the patient and choose the appropriate examination room. Make sure the environment going into the room is calm and not hurried. Keeping the patient comfortable and at ease is most important.

- *What about privacy?* The quality of your patient interactions depends on how comfortable the patient is. Respecting a patient's privacy can make him feel more comfortable. Drawing curtains around an examination table or bed, making sure the door is closed, and asking sensitive questions quietly help keep the patient at ease.

Communicating with Older Adults

You'll be faced with many unique challenges in your interactions with **geriatric**, or older adult patients. As medical technology improves, people are living longer. With this increase in the geriatric population comes a wide variety of types of patients within the older adult population itself. One older adult patient

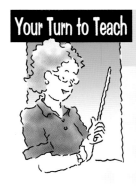

Your Turn to Teach

GETTING THE HEALTH CARE MESSAGE ACROSS TO ADULTS

Adult patients lead busy lives. Many patients may be so overwhelmed with everyday responsibilities that their health takes a backseat to the demands of their daily lives. Your own good health and cheerful attitude serves as an example for all patients to admire and follow. Use the following tips under direct instruction from a physician to help educate adult patients about ways to prevent future illness and maintain good health.

- *Diet.* Encourage patients to eat a balanced diet. Learn about the patient's food preferences, restrictions, and cultural background. Share your favorite market for buying the freshest produce. Keep a file of food pyramid pamphlets and healthy recipes that you can share with interested patients.

- *Exercise.* Remind patients about the importance of regular exercise. Emphasize to patients that even a 10-minute walk helps the body stay healthy. Share some fun exercises for patients who must sit for long periods. Encourage the patient to seek out or start an office walking group.

- *Hobbies.* Ask patients about any hobbies they might have. Find out what they do in their spare time. If they have little spare time, find out what they wish they could do if they had more spare time. Keep a file of local resources for patients to learn more about things that interest them.

- *Water.* Encourage patients to drink enough water every day. If the patient does not already do so, suggest he carry a personal water bottle. Adults should produce between one and two liters of urine each day. Adults are often dehydrated without knowing it.

might be bound to a wheelchair, hard of hearing, and suffering from dementia. Another older adult patient might be juggling hobbies, daily walks with friends, family time, and her upcoming trip to Europe. You might be surprised to find that many of your geriatric patients have more active social lives than most of your adult or adolescent patients!

The one common factor shared by all geriatric patients is their age. But age is not necessarily a limiting factor for all patients of this group. Because of this, your challenge as a medical assistant is to treat each geriatric patient as an individual, but always keep in mind the issues that go along with advancing age.

OLDER ADULTHOOD

You might refer to patients in the later stages of adulthood by different names—older adults, senior citizens, or the geriatric set. The older adult patient may experience a number of health-related issues. Loss of memory, loss of hearing, decreased mobility, and weakened vision are a few of these issues. Some geriatric patients may experience any or all of these in varying degrees.

The lifestyle of the older adult also varies from individual to individual. Many older adults may live either in a nursing home, assisted living complex, or alone. But many also live with their families, with partners, or with roommates.

Along with the realities faced by older adults are the many myths that exist. Because of these myths, some health care practitioners may not treat older adults with the respect and dignity

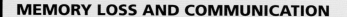

Listen to This   **MEMORY LOSS AND COMMUNICATION**

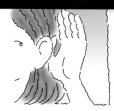

It's not uncommon for an older adult patient to suffer from some memory loss. If you know that a patient has this problem, here are some tips you can use to make your interaction with the patient positive and effective:

- Write instructions in easy-to-understand terms. Use simple words.
- Use large printed letters. Use ink that is easy to see.
- Have the patient repeat what you wrote. This helps reinforce the information.
- If applicable, ask the patient to show you how he will perform a procedure. This also helps reinforce what the patient must remember.
- Make a large appointment calendar for the patient. Write in medication times, therapy appointments, physician appointments, and any other health-related information on the calendar. Have the patient cross off each task as it's completed.

they deserve. Check the list of myths below to see how many of your own ideas about older adults look familiar.

- Old people are weak and sick.
- Old people can no longer learn.
- Old people are boring.
- Old people are always lonely.
- Old people have lost interest in life.
- Old people do everything slowly.
- Old people can't be trusted to make rational decisions.

All of the statements above have one thing in common—they are all false. How many of these myths are part of your attitude toward older adults? The more older adult patients you treat, the more you'll discover that individuals within this age group are as varied as those within any other age group.

SPEAKING EFFECTIVELY WITH OLDER ADULTS

Although each older adult patient should be treated as an individual, it's important that you recognize some issues common to this age group:

- Many older adult patients may have chronic health problems that have become part of their lifestyles. These chronic conditions must be considered when treating new ailments or conditions.
- Many older adult patients fear a decline in their good health. For many older adults, the loss of their good health means a loss of independence. Having to depend more and more on others is difficult.
- Many older adults fear death. As seniors get older, family members and friends pass on, and the reality of death becomes clearer. Encourage older patients to stay busy and to socialize often. This will help them continue to live full and active lives and to think less about death.

As a medical assistant, you want to make your communications with older adult patients as effective as possible. Along with the issues listed above, keep the following communication goals in mind when speaking with older adults.

Restore the Person's Sense of Control

When you first greet an older adult patient, introduce yourself. Ask the patient what name she prefers to be called. Keep the conversation cheerful and positive. Use humor when appropriate

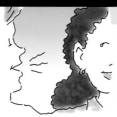

Send and Receive

SHATTERING MYTHS ABOUT OLDER ADULTS

Allowing myths about older adults to affect the way you interact and communicate with these patients creates a barrier to effective therapeutic communication. As with patients of any age group, you must learn what the older adult patient's needs are. This is essential to developing effective communication channels with this population.

Here is an example of an ineffective and effective dialogue between a medical assistant and an older adult patient. As you read through the dialogue, see if you can spot any of the myths listed above.

Imagine you're meeting Mr. Currie for the first time. Mr. Currie is 75-years-old and is experiencing pain in his chest each time he finishes a meal.

Ineffective:

- "Hello, Mr. Currie. What brings you here today?" You speak more loudly and slowly than usual, assuming Mr. Currie can't hear.

- You proceed to ask Mr. Currie some general questions about his symptoms and general health. You decide to skip the health history questions, assuming Mr. Currie won't be able to answer them.

- "Let me help you onto this examination table, Mr. Currie." You assume Mr. Currie can't get onto the table by himself.

As you have already learned, not all older adult patients are hard of hearing. Nor do all older adult patients have trouble remembering details or events. Regardless of the patient's age, you should always ask if the patient would like assistance getting up onto the examination table. Never assume a patient needs help. But always ask, out of courtesy and respect, if a patient would like some assistance. If you suspect a patient can't hear you, ask the patient if he understands what you have just said.

Effective:

- "Hello, Mr. Currie. What brings you here today?" You greet Mr. Currie in a normal voice. Mr. Currie replies that he is having some pain in his chest after he eats.

- You proceed to ask Mr. Currie about his general health history. Mr. Currie remembers all but one or two dates of past surgeries.

- "Mr. Currie, I'd like to have you get up onto the examination table. Would you like me to help you?"

As with all patients, be aware of any verbal and nonverbal clues the older adult patient gives you. When in doubt, ask the patient if he has had any difficulty in hearing what you have said. Ask if the patient needs assistance. Ask if the patient has any questions. In this regard, the older adult patient is no different from any patient of any other age group.

and possible. Involve the patient in the decision-making process.

Some older adult patients respond well to routine and structure. For these patients, appointments on the same day of the week at the same time are easier to remember. A regular appointment that is always at 2 P.M. on Monday is easier to remember than an appointment that keeps changing. Help older patients maintain their sense of independence by making it easier to take control of their health care.

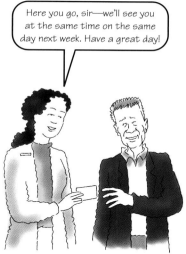

Here you go, sir—we'll see you at the same time on the same day next week. Have a great day!

Pace of Communication

Some older patients may not be able to understand what you say if you speak too quickly. Some patients may get impatient if you speak too slowly. As you get to know each older adult patient, learn the best ways to communicate with him. Be aware of any hearing, vision, or mental impairments your patient may have. Look for verbal and nonverbal clues that tell you if the patient understands and follows what you say. Decide what communication skills work best for each patient. With time, you'll begin to tailor your communication style to each patient.

Also keep in mind that some older adult patients may need more time for their appointments. Adding an extra 15 minutes to the appointment will prevent having to rush the patient.

Respect and Dignity

Treat all patients with respect and dignity. Older adult patients deserve your respect. Along with your respect, keep in mind the patient's need for quiet and privacy. Here are some tips for respecting patients during an office visit:

- Use the name the patient prefers, especially with older patients.
- Ask permission before performing all procedures.
- Take time to explain to the patient the steps of every procedure.
- Encourage the patient to ask questions. Make sure any questions for the physician are delivered to the physician.

Simple courtesies such as saying "please" and "thank you" also help show your respect for the patient.

Reassurance

One of the most important communication skills you can use with any patient is being able to sense when a patient becomes fearful or confused. A patient's expression or body language may tell you that he needs to be reassured or comforted. Or the patient may just tell you, "I'm confused," or "I do not understand." When this happens, take time to soothe the patient. Find out exactly what the patient is confused or upset about, and then address the issue specifically.

Cue Detection

As you can probably see by now, the ability to sense a patient's nonverbal cues is an important key in your ability to communicate effectively. This skill is called **cue detection.** Some of these cues are easy to spot. Others take time and experience to observe. Not all patients will tell you when they do not understand something you have said. They might feel embarrassed to admit they do not understand. Instead, you must look for the nonverbal clues that signal their confusion.

- The patient may look away when he gets confused.
- The patient might blankly say, "That's fine," or "All right."
- The patient may suddenly change the subject or want to leave.

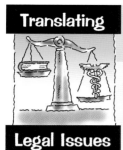

Translating

Legal Issues

LEGAL AND NONLEGAL ISSUES FOR OLDER ADULTS

Older adult patients face several difficult issues, legal and nonlegal, as they approach the end of their lives. Although you're not an attorney, you still have a responsibility to emphasize to patients the importance of addressing these issues. Nonlegal issues include:

- *Being ignored.* Many older adult patients fear that their pain will be ignored. They also fear that their pain is the sign of a debilitating illness. As a result, the patient may be afraid to admit that he is in pain. Or the patient may put off seeing a physician, hoping the pain will go away.

- *Dying alone.* Some older adults fear they will die alone and in misery. This may prevent some patients from being able to sleep restfully or from being able to discuss these fears with others.

- *Paying for health care.* Many seniors fear they will not be able to afford expensive medical care or medications. Many older adult patients may have limited financial resources for long-term health care.

These nonlegal issues are a source of stress and concern for older adult patients.

There are several legal issues that should also be addressed.

- *Do not resuscitate (DNR) order.* This order is placed by a patient's physician in the patient's medical file and states that cardiopulmonary resuscitation should not be performed.

- *Living will (one kind of advance directive).* This is a legal document that a person draws up while the patient is still capable of making decisions for her own health care. The document describes a person's health care preferences.

- *Durable power of attorney for health care (another kind of advance directive).* This is a legal document that names a specific person to make decisions about the patient's health care should the patient no longer be able to make decisions for herself.

Encourage older adult patients to discuss all of these issues with their family members and with the physician. Emphasize the importance of addressing these issues before it's too late. Try to provide patients with a resource list with phone numbers, addresses, or e-mail addresses of professionals, such as attorneys, who can help them with these legal issues.

Your cue detection skills will be a valuable tool in strengthening the communications you have with older adult patients.

Empathy

Empathy is being able to identify with the way another person feels. Being able to empathize with the concerns of your older adult patients will help you greatly in your communications with them. Being empathetic means you're sensitive to each patient's feelings and problems. Be sure to carry your empathy over to family and friends of the patient. A simple statement such as, "This must be a hard time for you. How are you doing?" sends a message of sincerity and caring.

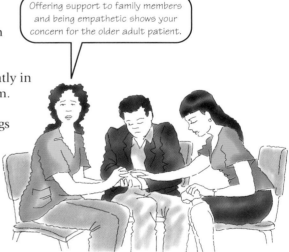
Offering support to family members and being empathetic shows your concern for the older adult patient.

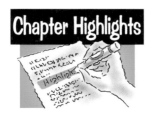
Chapter Highlights

- Humans grow and develop in different ways throughout their lives. Biological, social, and psychological factors affect this process.
- Piaget's cognitive development theory states that learning is based on interaction with your environment.
- Freud describes three major forces as the id (instincts), ego (reality and reason), and superego (the ideal self).

- Freud's reality principle states that the ego takes care of a need as soon as an appropriate object is found.

- Freud's pleasure principle is used to describe the primary function of the id—to decrease pain and increase pleasure.

- Erikson's eight psychosocial crises, or tasks, are: trust versus mistrust; autonomy versus shame and doubt; initiative versus guilt; industry versus inferiority; identity versus role confusion; intimacy versus isolation; generativity versus stagnation; and ego integrity versus despair.

- The principle of mutuality refers to the interaction of generations. Parents influence their children's development, and in turn children influence their parents' development.

- Operant conditioning is based on the principle that rewarded behavior will be repeated and that unrewarded behavior will not be repeated. According to this theory, the reinforcement a person receives after performing an action will determine whether that person repeats that action in the future.

- A knowledge of developmental theories will help you communicate effectively with patients of different ages and at various stages of development. This knowledge will also help you understand patients' behavior patterns and how these patterns may affect their health.

- A holistic approach to health care treats the whole patient, not just the condition.

- When communicating with children, your words, tone, and body language are important. Talk at eye level, speak gently, move slowly and visibly, announce your touch, rephrase often, allow crying, and use toys when appropriate.

- When communicating with adolescents, respect their privacy, and give them choices. Stay open, honest, and respectful. Use "I" messages to keep blame and judgmental statements out of the conversation.

- When communicating with adults, consider their life experience and lifestyle. Assess how much information the adult patient wants to know and make sure your messages are clear. Make sure the adult patients can follow their treatment plans.

- When communicating with older adults, remember that this population is diverse. Treat older adult patients with respect and dignity and involve them in decision making. Look for verbal and nonverbal cues and provide reassurance and empathy when appropriate.

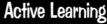

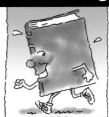

PART 1: MAKING OBSERVATIONS

Find a public area and observe one person's behavior for several minutes. Try to determine that person's stage of development. If this individual were a patient, assess how his stage of development would affect your communication with him. Take notes explaining the adaptations to communication you could make based on your assessment.

PART 2: PUTTING IT INTO PRACTICE

Divide into groups of four. On four pieces of paper, write the name of one of the four age groups: child, adolescent, adult, older adult. Using four pieces of a different-colored paper, write one of four medical conditions: fever, skin rash, cough, ear infection. Fold all eight pieces of paper and place them into a box or container.

Next, have two people from each group choose one of each colored paper. These two group members will play the part of patients; the other two group members will act as medical assistants. In turns, each patient/medical assistant pair will act out a brief scenario in which the "patient" attempts to describe his illness and the "medical assistant" adjusts her communication style according to the patient's age group. After both pairs have acted out their scenarios, discuss within your group the ways in which the "medical assistants" had to adjust their communication for each "patient."

Chapter 4

BUILDING BRIDGES: COMMUNICATING WITH PATIENTS

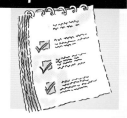

Chapter Checklist

- Describe the components of the patient interview
- Use open-ended and closed-ended questions and indirect statements to gather information from patients
- Identify the challenges to communication
- Explain the defense mechanisms employed by patients
- Use problem-solving skills
- Describe legal and ethical communication issues
- Explain the importance of confidentiality

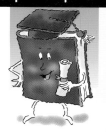

Chapter Competencies

- Interview effectively (ABHES Competency 2.f.)
- Be attentive, listen, and learn (ABHES 2.a.)
- Recognize and respond to verbal and nonverbal communication (ABHES Competency 2.i., 2.k., and 2.l.; CAAHEP Competency 3.c.1.b. and 3.c.1.c.)
- Obtain and record a patient history (ABHES Competency 4.a.; CAAHEP Competency 3.b.4.c.)
- Be impartial and show empathy when dealing with patients (ABHES Competency 2.b.)
- Be cognizant of ethical boundaries (ABHES Competency 1.d.)
- Perform within legal and ethical boundaries (CAAHEP Competency 3.c.2.b.)

- Demonstrate knowledge of federal and state health care legislation and regulations (CAAHEP Competency 3.c.2.e.)
- Monitor legislation related to current health care issues and practices (ABHES Competency 5.g.)
- Maintain confidentiality at all times (ABHES Competency 1.b.)
- Identify and respond to issues of confidentiality (CAAHEP Competency 3.c.2.a.)
- Use appropriate guidelines when releasing records or information (ABHES Competency 5.c.)
- Follow established policy in initiating or terminating medical treatment (ABHES Competency 5.d.)

Communicating with patients is a process that requires more than simply listening and speaking. To communicate effectively, you need to develop the right skills and put them into practice. This chapter will help you learn how to communicate effectively with different types of patients. You'll also learn the appropriate procedures and practices to use when dealing with patients. Communication skills are exercised in every aspect of medical assisting, so learning to use them well will help you succeed at work!

Patient Interviews

There are a variety of reasons that patients visit the physician, whether they have a specific ailment or they just need an annual check-up. Part of your job as a medical assistant is to gather information from patients to find out why they are visiting the medical office. Patient interviews are conducted to collect the patient's current and past medical information. The interview can also help the physician assess the patient's health care concerns and make a diagnosis.

The *new patient interview* occurs when the patient arrives for his first office visit. The purpose of this interview is to gather and record initial information, such as the patient's medical history and any current illnesses or conditions. This information gives the physician a picture of the patient's overall medical health.

For patients who have seen the physician before, an *established patient interview* is conducted. In this interview, the patient

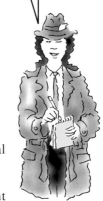

New patient interviews help you get all the facts about patients who haven't seen the physician before.

answers specific questions to determine his current health condition. This information will help the physician make the proper diagnosis and create a treatment plan after an examination has been completed.

The interview process includes three important steps:

1. creating the interview environment
2. identifying the patient's chief complaint, or reason for the office visit
3. helping the physician resolve the patient's chief complaint

CREATING THE RIGHT ENVIRONMENT

As a medical assistant, it will be your responsibility to create and maintain a professional interview environment. During an interview, a patient will often be asked to share information that is personal or confidential. Therefore, it's important to let the patient know that you're trustworthy and competent. A professional attitude and environment will make a patient feel comfortable opening up to you.

Professional Manner and Image

Your physical appearance makes the first impression on a patient, so it's important to look and sound your best. Here are some suggestions to consider when making the first impression.

- Practice good personal hygiene.
- Make sure your uniform is neat and clean.
- Introduce yourself and greet the patient with a smile.
- Be patient and sensitive as patients recall their personal medical information.

A positive and respectful attitude will go a long way in establishing good rapport, or good relationships, with patients.

Watch Your Tone

Communication involves not only *what* you say, but *how* you say it. Tone of voice helps the listener understand the message you're trying to convey. You want the message you send a patient to be a positive one. When conducting a patient interview, speak in a calm, pleasant tone of voice. Remember to control your volume and pitch. A monotone voice might indicate to the patient that you're bored or uninterested in the interview process. But a professional tone of voice shows a patient that you care about her health care.

Office Space

The medical office should have a positive and professional atmosphere. The waiting room should be neat and comfortable. Excessive noise or a crowded area might make a patient feel stressed.

Once you're ready to conduct the interview, take the patient into a private office or examination room. Conducting the interview in a private room ensures that other patients or staff members won't overhear the patient's private medical concerns. It may also help the patient feel more comfortable sharing this information with you.

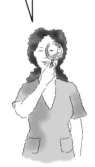

Use proper interviewing skills to help the physician *identify* the patient's problem.

IDENTIFYING THE PATIENT'S PROBLEM

The medical information you gather during the patient interview will help the physician identify the patient's problem. You can gather thorough and accurate information by:

- using proper interviewing skills
- paying attention to each interview component
- asking proper questions

Interviewing Skills

As a medical assistant, you'll need to learn and use the communication skills that will help you conduct a proper and thorough patient interview. Effective interviewing involves:

- being aware of the messages you're sending
- listening actively
- letting the patient know that you've understood his message

Using proper interview skills will help you obtain accurate and thorough information, which will help the physician make the correct diagnosis and prescribe appropriate treatment.

What We Say . . . or Do Not Say

Have you ever raised your eyebrows in amazement? Have you patted someone on the back as a form of encouragement? We all have nonverbal ways of expressing ourselves. But did you know that these expressions are forms of communication? Whether you're aware of it or not, you're communicating messages to other people all the time.

There are so many different ways we communicate with one another. As you learned in Chapter 1, verbal communication is when people send and receive messages using words or language. It's usually the initial form of contact. Speaking to a patient about his health insurance policy is an example of verbal communication. Nonverbal communication, which you also read about in Chapter 1, involves exchanging messages without using words. It's frequently referred to as **body language** because your body does most of the talking! The following are examples of nonverbal communication:

- *Body position.* Turn your body toward a patient to give her your full attention.
- *Facial expressions.* A smile can communicate friendliness, and a concerned expression can let a patient know that you care about how she's feeling.
- *Touch.* A touch on the arm or a pat on the shoulder can be reassuring to a patient who seems nervous or anxious.
- *Gestures.* Hand movements can help you emphasize a point or convey your interest in the topic being discussed.

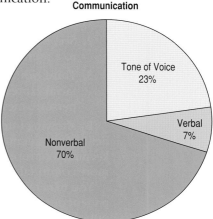

As you can see, nonverbal messages (body language) make up a big piece of the communication pie.

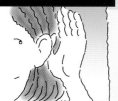

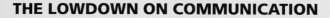

Listen to This   THE LOWDOWN ON COMMUNICATION

- How you say something with your tone and body language will affect the message—so make it positive!
- Be aware of the message your body language is sending. Body language includes body position, facial expressions, touch, and gestures.
- Your verbal communication should match your nonverbal communication. If you tell a patient that you care about his health concerns, but you're constantly glancing at the clock while he's talking, then you're sending mixed messages! Be consistent in thought and action.
- Remember to be friendly but professional. Chatting with a patient is fine, but discussing your personal problems is not. When communicating in the medical office, your focus should always be on the patients and their health needs.

I Hear You!

When interviewing patients, it's important to use active listening skills. But keep in mind that listening actively requires more than simply waiting quietly while another person speaks.

Active listening requires three things.

1. First, you must be engaged with what the other person is saying.

2. Second, you need to be attentive. Try to keep interruptions to a minimum and give the speaker your full attention.

3. Third, you need to be observant. Nonverbal clues, such as facial expressions and gestures, can help you understand a person's message.

By showing interest in what a patient is saying, you'll help her feel confident that your main concern is with her. Also, keeping interruptions to a minimum can help patients feel more comfortable discussing their private health information.

You may receive many verbal and nonverbal clues from the patient during the interview process. Sometimes, the first words out of a patient's mouth are not necessarily the best clues as to her condition. For this reason, do not jump to conclusions at the beginning of an interview. You should wait until you have completed the entire interview process and all appropriate procedures before you draw any conclusions. Premature judgments can have a negative impact on the communication process between you and the patient. Jumping to conclusions may also cause you to relay less important information to the physician, while ignoring more important details the physician should know.

Be a Mirror for the Message

Okay, now you know how to listen actively to patients. But how do you let patients know that you've heard and understood them? Reflecting and paraphrasing are two communication skills that can help you do this.

Reflecting is repeating what you've heard, using open-ended statements or questions. For example, you might say, "Mr. Miller, you were saying that when your neck hurts you . . ." Reflecting allows the patient to

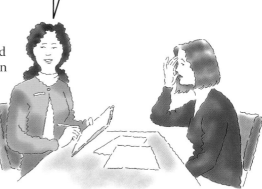

Pay attention to the patient's body language. Gestures and facial expressions can communicate important messages, too!

make further statements or clarify something you may not have understood. It also lets him know that you've listened and want to know more information.

Paraphrasing is restating what you've heard, using your own words. A paraphrased statement typically begins with, "What you're saying is . . ." or "It sounds like . . ." followed by the rephrased information. Paraphrasing lets the patient know that you've accurately understood what was said. It also allows the patient to clarify any misinterpretations you've made.

Interview Components

The patient interview includes several different components:

- the patient's medical history
- an assessment of the patient's signs and symptoms
- the patient's chief complaint and present illness
- documentation of the patient's history

Each component provides information the physician will use in diagnosing the patient and developing a treatment plan. That's why it's important to follow all of your office's policies and procedures when collecting information from a patient.

Medical History

The information gathered for a patient's medical history form is one of many documents in the medical office that is confidential and protected by a federal law called **Health Insurance Portability and Accountability Act of 1996 (HIPAA)**. (HIPAA is explained in more detail later in this chapter.) Only those who are directly involved with a patient's care may have access to the medical history form without the patient's consent.

Medical history forms may vary depending on the physician's practice specialty, but most forms include these elements:

- *Database.* This section includes the patient's name, address, and phone number. It also lists the appropriate contact information for the patient's employer and health insurance carrier. The patient's health insurance policy number, Social Security number, marital status, gender, and race are included in this section as well.

- *Past history (PH).* The patient's prior health status is recorded in this section. Information such as allergies, immunizations, childhood diseases, current and past medications, and previous illnesses, surgeries, and hospitalizations are typically found in this section.

- *Review of systems (ROS).* Included in this section is a full review of each of the body's systems (cardiovascular, respiratory, nervous, digestive, etc.). Specific questions, such as symptoms or known diseases for each system of the body, are included here.
- *Family history.* This section contains the health information of a patient's parents, siblings, and grandparents. This information is important because certain diseases or disorders are hereditary and more common in some families. If any immediate family member is deceased, the cause of death should be documented.
- *Social history.* The social history relates to the patient's lifestyle, such as marital status, occupation, education, and hobbies. It may also include information about a patient's diet and nutrition, alcohol and tobacco use, sexual history, or history of past abuse.

Assessing the Patient

During the interview, listen carefully to the patient as she describes her current health concerns to identify signs and symptoms. Identifying signs and symptoms will help you assess the patient's pre-existing conditions as well as potential health concerns.

Signs are objective information about a patient's health that can be observed by someone other than the patient. Some examples of signs include:

- rash
- bleeding
- coughing
- swelling
- vital sign measurements

Symptoms are subjective information about changes in health that are sensed by the patient. Symptoms aren't usually observable or measurable by people other than the patient. They include:

- headache
- neck pain
- nausea
- dizziness

Certain signs may indicate that a patient is experiencing some of these symptoms. For example, a patient who is wincing might be in pain, or a patient who is holding onto a railing might feel dizzy or need help walking. Pay attention to the outward signs so you'll know which action is best to take.

Chief Complaint and Present Illness

> Read the signs! A patient who is coughing might be experiencing symptoms such as sore throat or chest congestion.

After recording the patient's medical history and reviewing it for accuracy, you should find out why the patient has made an appointment to see the physician. Ask questions to gather information about the patient's *chief complaint* (CC). You might ask something like, "What's the reason for your visit today, Mr. Lin?" A simple question like this will open the lines of communication between you and the patient.

After determining the patient's chief complaint, you'll need to gather other details about the patient's *present illness* (PI). The present illness includes the order that symptoms occurred, as well as any medications the patient has taken. Remember to be tactful in your approach and allow the patient time to recall information and respond to your questions appropriately. (See *Types of Interview Questions.*)

Keep in mind that some patients may be visiting the office for routine examinations or tests. You'll still need to determine the chief complaint for these visits (e.g., annual physical examination), but there may not be additional information to gather regarding a present illness.

Documentation of Patient History

In some medical practices, medical assistants gather initial information from the patient using a list of interview questions. Other medical practices require the patient to complete a standard form before or during the first appointment. Patients who received the form in the mail are instructed to bring the completed form with them to the initial visit. In either case, you must check the form for completeness, as the physician will be using the information on the form to guide the examination.

In other offices, the physician may prefer to complete the entire form during the first in-office visit and examination. In this case, you should be familiar with the interview form and procedure so you may assist the physician.

TYPES OF INTERVIEW QUESTIONS

When you interview a patient, you'll need to use different types of questions to collect information. Varying your question style will help you gather the most accurate information. It will also allow the patient to describe her own health concerns and issues accurately.

Open-Ended Questions

You should use **open-ended questions** when seeking initial information about a patient's present illness. These questions encourage the patient to respond with more than one or two words. Open-ended questions often begin with the words:

- *how*
- *what*
- *when*
- *can*

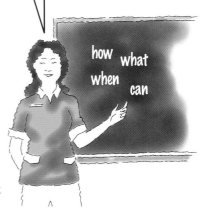

When asking open-ended questions, remember to use the key words *how, what, when,* and *can.*

For example, you might ask, "Can you please describe the symptoms you've been experiencing?" or "What medications have you taken for the pain?" Questions like these allow the patient to explain his problem in his own words.

When asking open-ended questions, avoid influencing a patient's answers. Instead of asking questions based on the symptoms you think a patient "should" be experiencing (based on his chief complaint), allow the patient to name and describe any symptoms he's feeling.

Closed-Ended Questions

Ask **closed-ended questions** when you need to gather more specific information. These questions can be answered with one word or phrase. They often begin with the words:

- *do*
- *is*
- *are*

For example, you might ask a patient, "Did the swelling in your leg start today?" or "Does the pain return every evening?" These closed-ended questions can be answered with a simple "yes" or "no."

Indirect Statements

Indirect statements are used to obtain a response without making the patient feel that she is being questioned. You might say to the patient, "Tell me more about your pain." This method of questioning allows the patient to volunteer additional information and clarify previous statements. You can also use indirect statements when a patient seems quiet or reserved, or if you feel that she is offering too little information.

RESOLUTION OF THE PATIENT'S PROBLEM

During the interview, you'll work to establish a lasting rapport with the patient. This rapport should extend to the resolution phase of the interviewing process. The following is a list of things to keep in mind when helping the patient resolve a health problem.

- Explain the problem in terms the patient can understand.
- Allow time for the patient to ask questions.
- Schedule a follow-up visit if requested by the physician.
- Have empathy for the patient instead of sympathy.
- Establish trust with the patient.

In Layman's Terms, Please

When explaining any problem, use words the patient can understand. It's okay to use appropriate medical terminology, but remember to adjust this information according to the patient's level of understanding and ask for feedback to make sure the patient understands what you're saying. For example, rather than telling the patient he had a myocardial infarction, you might explain instead that he had a heart attack, and then ask if he knows what this means. Using advanced medical terms might frighten or confuse the patient.

Question and Answer Time

Allow for questions. A patient will naturally be curious about her health care, and might have many questions regarding her problem. Be patient and take the time to answer all her questions to the best of your ability. It's okay if you do not know the answer to something. If you do not know the answer, have the physician or another qualified staff member talk with the patient.

Follow-Up

Provide for a follow-up visit. The physician may want to see the patient again to check on his progress. Talk with the physician to understand the best course of action to take. Then explain to the patient when he will need to come back to the office, if necessary.

Show Your Soft Side

Express warmth and understanding. A patient's diagnosis or prognosis may be upsetting, and the patient will need time and space to cope with this new information. It's important that you express to the patient your empathy, rather than your sympathy.

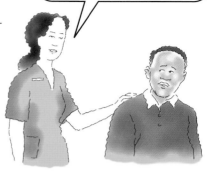

You appear to be worried about the procedure. Is there anything I can do to make this easier for you?

- **Empathy** is the ability to relate to and understand the patient's feelings. When you empathize with someone, you imagine how you would feel in her situation.
- **Sympathy** is feeling sorry or having pity for someone.

Empathy involves focusing on understanding how and why the patient feels the way she does, so that you can help her. Empathy helps you recognize the patient's emotions so that you can provide reassurance and comfort.

Establish Trust

Establish trust with the patient. After receiving news about a health problem, the patient may feel unsure or uncomfortable. Trust is about more than just keeping a patient's confidences. You must also earn the patient's trust by being sincere and respectful. A patient is more likely to be open and honest if he trusts the person conducting the interview.

Challenges to Communication

Communication can be a challenge when you're met with conversational road blocks. What might cause a road block in your communication with a patient? Language barriers and working with patients with special needs are just two of the communication challenges you might face. You need to have the professional skills and know-how to meet these challenges head-on. It's important to be prepared when communicating with patients who have special needs. The following information explains some of the situations that require specific communication skills and how to use those skills effectively when dealing with patients.

LANGUAGE BARRIERS

Effective communication relies upon the use of language, but what if a patient can't understand or speak English? In these situations, you'll need an interpreter to bridge the language gap between you and the patient. A staff member might serve as an interpreter, or a patient's English-speaking family member

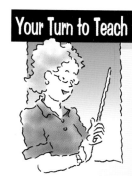

Your Turn to Teach

RESOLVING A PATIENT'S PROBLEM: FEVER

A patient who has a fever is most likely suffering from his body's natural response to disease and infection. A fever may be uncomfortable, but a high fever (above 101°F) can be dangerous and should be brought down to a lower temperature. The physician may ask you to teach a patient how to cope with a fever. You can help resolve the patient's problem by providing the following tips:

- Unless you're experiencing nausea and vomiting, drink clear fluids to keep body tissues hydrated.
- Make sure clothes and bed linens remain clean and dry, especially if the fever has caused sweating.
- Try to avoid becoming chilled. Chills cause shivering, which leads to a rise in body temperature.
- Eat a light diet (as tolerated) and be sure to give your body the rest it needs.
- Take antipyretics (drugs that reduce fever), but do not give medications containing aspirin to children under 18-years-old.
- Sometimes, the physician will prescribe antibiotics, depending on the type of infection. Take all medication that the physician prescribes as directed.

might be able to help. In either case, be sure that the interpreter fully understands the message you're intending to send.

Alternative Solutions

If a reliable interpreter isn't present, then a phrase book of common medical questions and possible answers may help you communicate. If your area has a large population of non–English-speaking patients, your office should be provided with at least one appropriate phrase book.

HEARING IMPAIRMENTS

There are many forms of hearing impairments, and they can range from partial hearing loss to *anacusis,* complete hearing loss. To communicate with patients who can't hear well or at

Listen to This

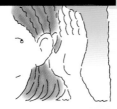

BRIDGING THE LANGUAGE GAP

The following are some suggestions for communicating with non–English-speaking patients.

- Do not shout. Raising your voice will not increase a patient's understanding.
- Gestures can sometimes help you clarify your message.
- If you're using an interpreter, speak directly to the patient with the interpreter in your line of sight, so that the patient can see your facial expressions. Never use a child as an interpreter.
- Speak slowly, using short and clear sentences that require simple answers. The patient may understand some English.
- Avoid using slang or other expressions (such as "It's raining cats and dogs") that may not translate well.
- Avoid distractions and provide the patient with a quiet, relaxed atmosphere.
- Learn some basic phrases of the most common languages spoken in your area. If you're able to say even short phrases, such as "good morning" or "please," patients will appreciate your effort.
- If you can speak a second language, your employer may ask you to complete a proficiency test showing that you can speak in medically accurate terms in your second language. After doing so, you may be allowed to act as an interpreter in your medical office.
- Choose an interpreter of the same sex as the patient. Some cultures do not allow discussion of body-related topics between members not of the same sex.

> Any time you communicate with anyone in the medical office, avoid using slang, especially when talking to non–English-speaking patients.

all, you need to have awareness and sensitivity to each patient's needs. These suggestions may help.

- Touch the patient gently to gain his attention.
- Talk directly to the patient, face to face. Some patients may read lips; others want to see your facial expressions.
- Talk to the patient in a well-lit area.

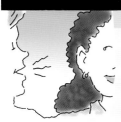

Send and Receive

BREAKING DOWN COMMUNICATION BARRIERS

Imagine that you're a medical assistant interviewing a patient who speaks very little English. What would you do? How would you communicate? Here are some examples of ineffective and effective dialogue.

Ineffective:

- "What brings you here today, Ms. Garcia?" Ms. Garcia looks puzzled. Speaking louder, the medical assistant repeats, "I said what brings you here today, Ms. Garcia?"

- "According to your chart, it looks like the physician treated you last month for a herniated intervertebral disk. Have you been experiencing unremitting pain or weakness in your extremities?"

When communicating with non–English-speaking patients, it's important to speak in simple sentences. When possible, avoid using advanced medical terminology. If a word or phrase may be confusing to English-speaking patients, imagine what it must sound like to patients who speak a completely different language altogether!

Effective:

- "What brings you here today, Ms. Garcia?" Ms. Garcia looks puzzled. "¿Cómo se siente?" (*How do you feel?*)

- "¿Tiéne dolor?" (*Do you have pain?*) Ms. Garcia nods. "Please point to the part of your body that hurts." Ms. Garcia looks confused. The medical assistant demonstrates what she means by pointing to the different parts of her own body or by using a chart.

If an interpreter isn't available, use a phrase book of common medical questions in the patient's native language. Translated materials are available from various sources. Web-based materials from federal and state government organizations or materials downloaded from health departments can be used for translation. If you're unable to translate a phrase or question, use gestures to get your message across. By taking the extra time to obtain accurate information from the patient, you'll help the physician provide the best possible treatment.

- Lower your pitch, but speak distinctly and with force. Higher pitches are frequently lost with nerve damage. Shouting usually does not help and might distort what could be heard.
- Use demonstrations when needed.
- Pictograms, or flash cards, may aid communication.
- Use short sentences and state your words clearly.
- Talk in a quiet, relaxed environment so that the patient isn't distracted.

If you're still unable to communicate effectively, consider using written communication instead. You can use a notepad to communicate messages back and forth, or a pamphlet may provide the necessary information. (Written communication will be discussed in more detail in Chapter 8.)

COGNITIVE IMPAIRMENTS

Cognitive impairments may influence a patient's ability to communicate effectively. Dementia, Alzheimer's disease, and cerebrovascular accidents are all examples of cognitive impairments because they affect the brain's ability to function and process information. The following is a list of suggestions to follow when communicating with cognitively impaired patients.

- Consult with the patient's caregiver or legal guardian. This individual may be responsible for making medical decisions for the patient.
- Create a distraction-free environment. There should be little or no background noise during the interview.
- Establish trust with the patient. Have patience and remember to be respectful at all times.
- Use closed-ended questions. You shouldn't require a patient to give long, complex responses. The patient should be able to answer most questions with a simple "yes" or "no."
- If the patient has to make a decision, start by offering a choice between two alternatives. Confusing the patient with multiple options may make him upset or angry.
- Provide positive feedback. Let the patient know that he is doing a good job during the interview process. Encourage and thank the patient for his cooperation and attention.

The Voice of Experience

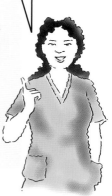

WORKING WITH SPECIAL-NEEDS PATIENTS

Q: *I'm new to the medical field. How do I work with a patient who has cognitive impairments?*

A: A patient with cognitive disabilities has different needs from other patients. In my experience, it's a good idea to talk with a spouse, relative, or whoever might have come with the patient on the visit. A relative who lives with the patient might have some tips for better communication.

Keep in mind that patients with cognitive impairments might forget who you are or become confused easily. Remind the patient who you are and reorient him to his surroundings when appropriate.

Above all, have patience with yourself! Every patient is different. Once you become familiar with a patient's needs, the communication process will go more smoothly.

> Remember, each patient is different! The same communication techniques might not work with every patient you meet.

COMMUNICATION BARRIERS

Non-therapeutic statements will close the lines of communication between you and the patient. Avoid the following:

- *Indifference.* Patients need to feel that you value their concerns. Indifference is often conveyed nonverbally by yawning, sighing, and eye rolling. These gestures will make a patient feel like you do not care about his health care needs.

- *Reassuring clichés.* These are careless and overused responses, such as, "Do not worry, you'll be okay." These statements can seem insincere and uninspired.

- *Advising.* These statements put the health care professional in control instead of the patient. You might have the best intentions, but statements that begin with "If I were you, I'd . . ." sound preachy and aggressive.

> Avoid setting up communication barriers—it's never a good idea to label patients or make sarcastic remarks.

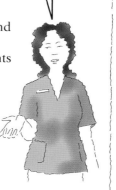

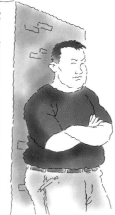

- *Criticizing.* These statements are never acceptable. Criticizing includes comments such as, "You should have come in yesterday, when you first began noticing the symptoms." These comments make the patient feel guilty and judged.

- *Denying.* A denying statement, such as "That can't be right," tells the patient he's wrong. This type of statement implies that the patient isn't telling the truth.

- *Lecturing.* Educating patients is important, but lecturing them isn't productive. Statements like, "I've told you several times now . . ." or "You know you really should . . ." are neither encouraging nor helpful.

- *Sarcasm.* These statements say one thing but imply another. Making a statement such as, "You must really like desserts" to a patient who is overweight will have a negative effect on the patient's emotional well-being. Making jokes at a patient's expense is never appropriate.

- *Changing the subject.* Changing the subject isn't conducive to providing quality care. It's important to listen to patients regardless of your personal feelings about the subject being discussed. If a patient has medical questions or concerns that you aren't qualified to answer, however, refer him to a physician.

Defense Mechanisms

The well-known neurologist Sigmund Freud developed the theory of **defense mechanisms**. He thought that people use defense mechanisms as tools to help them cope with their feelings. Some psychologists think that defense mechanisms are negative and limit a person's growth, while others think they help protect us. Individuals may consciously or unconsciously use defense mechanisms. The following sections describe common defense mechanisms and examples of each.

DENY, DENY, DENY

Denial is failing to acknowledge a problem, an experience, or a reality. A patient who is going through denial might say something like, "I do not have cancer. The lab must have sent the wrong results to my doctor."

BUT I DO NOT REMEMBER THAT . . .

Repression is a method of forgetting. It can also be described as "temporary amnesia." This defense mechanism may cause a person to forget an upsetting or traumatic experience. For example, a victim of child abuse might say, "I do not remember being physically abused as a child."

COMPENSATING FOR WEAKNESSES

A person who is attempting to make up for a real or imagined weakness or deficiency might use **compensation**. A patient might compensate for being overweight by saying, "I'm not overweight, I'm big-boned. That's why I'm so good at lifting heavy things. It helps me at my job."

DISPLACING ANGER

Displacement refers to shifting the angry emotions of a situation from a threatening to a nonthreatening object. An example of displacement would be an angry person's slamming a door instead of talking about his problem.

THE PROBLEM WITH PROJECTION

Someone who is using **projection** as a defense mechanism would attribute her own thoughts to another individual. For example, an angry patient might accuse you of being hostile toward her.

CANCEL THAT BEHAVIOR

Undoing is trying to cancel out a negative behavior. This defense mechanism provides a way of making amends for something you thought, said, or did. Having thoughts about harming someone and then being overly nice to that person can be a way of trying to "undo" your bad thoughts. For example, a person who abuses others may purchase gifts for the person he has abused as a way of making amends for his actions.

SOMEONE TO IDENTIFY WITH

A person who unconsciously copies another person's behavior to compensate for low self-esteem is using **identification**. An example of identification would be a mother who becomes anorexic because she wants to be thin like her young daughter.

REGRESSING BACK TO THE BEGINNING

Regression involves going back to an earlier stage of development. A child may begin to suck his thumb again or wet the bed when he is staying in the hospital for an illness.

RATIONALIZATION: NOT ALWAYS RATIONAL

Rationalization is a way of justifying one's behavior. A patient might rationalize her actions by saying, "Yes, I'm diabetic. But I exercised today, and I only had a few cookies. What harm could it do?"

SOCIALLY ACCEPTABLE BEHAVIOR IS SUBLIME

Sublimation is redirecting a socially unacceptable impulse into a socially acceptable behavior. For example, one reason a patient may give for playing football is that it's a good way to get out his anger or frustration.

Problem-Solving Skills

As a medical assistant, you'll play a role in the problem-solving process. Problem solving is a process that includes five key steps.

1. Identify the problem.
2. Develop a treatment plan.
3. Implement the plan.
4. Evaluate the results.
5. Maintain or modify the plan.

It's important to follow office guidelines and procedures when participating in patient care. If you're ever confused or unsure about something regarding a patient's health, you should consult the physician.

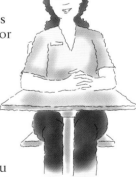

Problem-solving skills aren't just for math class! These skills will help you provide better patient care.

IDENTIFY THE PROBLEM

What is the patient's present illness and chief complaint? It's your job to determine both of these during the patient interview. Then, a physician's examination will help determine the cause of the problem. Here are some questions you may ask the patient about his symptoms to identify the patient's chief complaint.

- What are your symptoms?
- Are you experiencing any pain? If so, where?
- When are your symptoms worse?
- Have you taken any medication to help alleviate the symptoms?
- Do you have any symptoms or signs that indicate a medical emergency?

DEVELOP A TREATMENT PLAN

Once the physician has identified the problem, she'll need to decide on a treatment plan. You may work with the physician to create an appropriate treatment plan for the patient. The physician will consider the following:

- How serious is the condition?
- Does this patient need medication or other pharmaceuticals? If so, what is the prescribed dosage?
- Should this patient change an aspect of his lifestyle, such as nutrition and exercise habits, sexual health, or activity level?
- Should this patient see a psychiatrist, surgeon, or other medical professional?
- Does the patient need any further tests or procedures?

IMPLEMENT THE PLAN

Patient education can be a big part of your job as a medical assistant. Once the physician has developed a treatment plan, it may be your job to explain this plan to the patient. Here are some tips for helping this education process run smoothly.

- Explain the treatment plan to the patient and include the reasons for taking this course of action.
- Allow time for questions.
- Let the patient know what he can do to improve his health condition and what types of treatments he will be required to follow.
- Ask for feedback to be sure the patient thoroughly understands each component of the treatment plan and how the treatment might change or affect his current lifestyle or health.
- Discuss and plan for any necessary follow-up appointments or treatments.

EVALUATE THE RESULTS

After the patient has implemented the treatment plan, the physician will usually wait for a period of time before evaluating whether the treatment plan was effective. You may be asked to phone the patient a few days after the patient's office visit to find out how the treatment is progressing. During this call or during the patient's next appointment, you may help the physician determine the patient's response to the plan by addressing these questions.

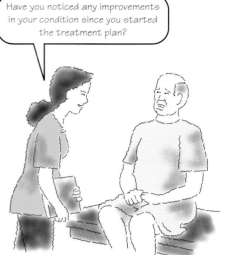

Have you noticed any improvements in your condition since you started the treatment plan?

- Has the patient been following the prescribed treatment plan?
- Is he feeling better?
- Has his condition improved or worsened?
- Have any new symptoms developed?

The physician will further evaluate the patient to determine whether the treatment is working and whether further treatment or changes to treatment are necessary.

MAINTAIN OR MODIFY THE PLAN

After obtaining information from the patient, the physician will use the information and observations you've gathered to help determine whether or not the treatment plan should be maintained or modified. The physician will consider the following:

- Should the treatment plan be modified to fit the patient's lifestyle better?
- Is the patient taking prescribed medication as directed?
- Has the medication achieved the desired effect?
- Has the patient noticed or reported any side effects from the medication?

The physician is responsible for deciding whether to maintain or modify a patient's treatment plan. However, you'll often be required to reinforce the details and consequences of the physician's decision with the patient.

Legal and Ethical Issues

Legal and ethical issues will affect your communication with patients as well. To protect yourself and your employer, it's important to know what the law says about:

- patient confidentiality
- advance directives
- informed consent

THE HEALTH INSURANCE PORTABILITY AND ACCOUNTABILITY ACT

As you read earlier in the chapter, HIPAA is a federal law passed in 1996 to protect privacy and other health care rights for patients. HIPAA has four main objectives:

- ensuring health insurance portability for all people
- reducing health care fraud and abuse
- enforcing standards of health information
- guaranteeing security and privacy of health information

According to HIPAA, patients have the right to:

- request copies of their health records
- update their health records
- obtain a list of the disclosures a health care company has made (other than routine disclosures of patient information for the purposes of treatment, payment, and health care operations)
- request a restriction on certain uses or disclosures of their health information
- choose how to receive health information

Covered Entities

HIPAA defines physicians and health care facilities as *covered entities*. This means any patient information they transmit—whether it's oral, written, or electronic—is protected under federal law.

Covered Transactions

When two covered entities exchange patient information electronically by following HIPAA standards, it's called a *covered transaction*. In the medical office, most covered transactions will be made through the use of computers.

Although computers can provide a fast and easy way to transmit information, certain measures must be taken to secure the privacy of all patients. To maintain patients' security, health care professionals are urged to do the following:

- Keep all computer backup discs in a safe place away from patient areas.
- Store discs in a bank safe-deposit box.
- Use passwords that include characters other than letters and encrypt the passwords.

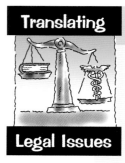

Translating

Legal Issues

HIPAA RULES!

The following is a list of legal issues to keep in mind regarding HIPAA policies and procedures for the medical office.

- There are specific guidelines to follow when sending information electronically. For example, protected patient information should be encrypted before it's e-mailed. Many software programs can help medical offices comply with these regulations.

- Medical offices must take appropriate steps to ensure that any company they communicate with also follows HIPAA regulations. This applies to health insurance companies, laboratories, other health care facilities, etc.

- Each medical practice must designate a privacy officer. This person is responsible for maintaining the privacy and security of all patients and making sure the office complies with HIPAA regulations.

- If a health institution wants to release a patient's health information for purposes other than treatment, payment, and routine health care operations, the patient must be asked to sign an authorization. Otherwise, the patient has the right to take legal action against the institution.

- Change computer login codes and other passwords every 30 days.

- Prepare a backup plan in the event that the computer system stops functioning.

- Keep computer screens out of the patients' view.

- Keep the fax machines and printers that receive protected patient information in a private place.

- Ensure that each user is restricted to the information needed to do his job.

- Create a written confidentiality policy that employees must sign. Include disciplinary consequences for breaches of confidentiality.

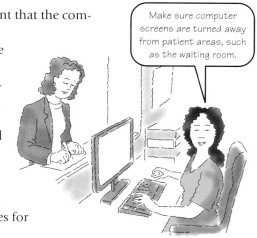

Make sure computer screens are turned away from patient areas, such as the waiting room.

- Train employees on their responsibilities regarding patient confidentiality. Training is available from vendors of medical software.
- Conduct routine audits that track each employee's movements through the electronic medical record (EMR) system.

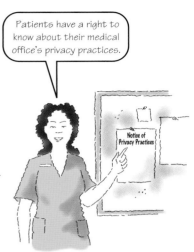

Patients have a right to know about their medical office's privacy practices.

Privacy Practices

A **Notice of Privacy Practices** is a written document that gives the details of a health care provider's privacy practices. According to HIPAA regulations, the medical office must post a note in all waiting room areas that explains the office's privacy practices. Policies and procedures must ensure that patients' safety and confidentiality are protected.

Protected Health Information

Protected health information is data about a patient's past, present, or future medical treatment that contain one or more *patient identifiers.* Examples of patient identifiers include:

- name
- date of birth
- Social Security number
- address
- phone number
- occupation
- age

This information is personal and should never be shared with anyone outside the medical practice without the patient's consent. All medical forms pertaining to a patient's health information are protected under HIPAA regulations. No one except those who are directly involved in a patient's care may have access to this information without the patient's permission. However, health information that has had all patient identifiers removed, or *de-identified information,* is not considered protected health information.

ADVANCE DIRECTIVES

In 1991, Congress passed the Self-Determination Act, which gives all hospitalized patients the right to make their own health care decisions as soon as they are admitted to the hospital. These decisions are referred to as **advance directives**. An advance directive is a statement of a person's wishes prior to a critical event, such as a health emergency.

Today, the medical community encourages patients to become actively involved in their own end-of-life decisions. Patients can even complete advance directives online. Advance directives can include special wishes, including whether a patient will accept or decline the use of a ventilator or feeding tube. Filling out an advance directive online is convenient, but it's important to make family members aware of these wishes to ensure that the wishes are carried out. The patient's next of kin should keep a copy of the directive, and another copy should be placed in the patient's medical record.

INFORMED CONSENT

The physician is responsible for obtaining the patient's informed consent whenever the treatment involves an invasive procedure or potential for risk, such as surgery. **Informed consent** is the patient's right to receive all information related to his condition. He can use this information to make a decision about having a certain procedure or treatment. Informed consent is also based on the patient's right to know every possible benefit, risk, or alternative to the suggested treatment before he makes a decision and the possible or likely outcome if no treatment is followed.

A consent form must include the following information:

- name of the procedure to be performed
- name of the physician who will perform the procedure
- name of the person who will administer anesthesia (if applicable)
- any potential risks from the procedure
- anticipated result or benefit from the procedure
- alternatives to the procedure and their risks
- likely effect on the patient's health if the procedure isn't performed
- any exclusions or specifications the patient requests
- statement indicating that all the patient's questions regarding the procedure have been answered
- patient's and witnesses' signatures and the date

As a medical assistant, you'll frequently witness consent signatures. The patient must voluntarily give his consent and understand the meaning of his decision. You and the physician will be responsible for communicating these issues to the patient.

Confidentiality

Confidentiality is respecting privileged information. Privileged information is held confidential within a protected relationship, such as the relationship between patient and physician. All information about patients is considered private or confidential, including written documents, computer files, and spoken information. Here are some tips to remember when protecting patient confidentiality:

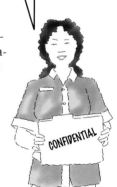

Remember, a patient's medical information is confidential! As a medical assistant, it's your duty to make sure private patient information does not get into the wrong hands.

- Never disclose information to any third party (such as an insurance company or a patient's family member) without the patient's consent.
- Patient information may be shared with consulting physicians or specialists without the patient's written authorization, as long as the physician is directly involved with the patient's care.
- When talking on the phone, avoid using the patient's name if others in the room may overhear.
- Never leave medical charts in an area where other patients or visitors may see them.
- Inform all new employees of confidentiality policies and procedures.

Releasing Information and Initiating or Terminating Treatment

Medical offices must establish policies that list the procedures for releasing patient records and initiating and terminating treatment.

RELEASING PATIENT INFORMATION

Although the physical medical record belongs to the physician, the information it contains belongs to the patient. For this reason, the patient (or the patient's legal guardian) must authorize any release of records.

Insurance companies, lawyers, other health care practitioners, and patients themselves may request copies of medical

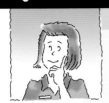

Say it Isn't So

DO FAMILY MEMBERS HAVE A RIGHT TO KNOW?

Is it ever acceptable to release a patient's diagnosis to a family member without the patient's consent?

Suppose you answer the phone and the woman on the other end of the line asks a question concerning another patient's medical history. She claims that she is the patient's wife and would like to know if he has any sexually transmitted diseases. She tells you that the patient refuses to take an STD test. You understand her concern and feel bad for her. Should you release this information?

Absolutely not! The patient hasn't given his permission to release this information. Do not let your personal feelings about a situation affect your judgment. You should tell the woman on the phone that you're not allowed to release that information, and she should talk to the patient directly about his sexual health history. She can also consult with her primary physician about her health concerns.

records. All requests should be made in writing and contain the following information:

- patient's name
- address
- Social Security number
- original signature

As you read earlier in the chapter, HIPAA now allows medical records to be released to specialists or other health care practitioners without the patient's signed authorization. However, the specialist or physician must be directly involved in the patient's care. HIPAA also allows patients to sign a waiver to have their medical information sent to their health insurance company for billing purposes. After the patient signs the waiver, all future billing information may be sent to the patient's insurance provider.

When releasing a medical record, provide a copy only. Never release the original medical record, except when ordered to do so by a court of law.

Subpoenas

A patient's medical record is a legal document. Lawyers may request medical records to submit as evidence in legal cases. Medical records can also be *subpoenaed,* or required by a court order, in cases such as malpractice lawsuits. In such situations, the patient's authorization is waived.

If an original medical record is subpoenaed, the physician may ask the judge to sign a document stating that he will temporarily take charge of the medical record. This signed document should be filed in the medical office until the document is returned. To further ensure the record's protection, a staff member may transport the original record to court on the day it's requested, and then return it to the medical office at the end of the court session.

Legally Required Disclosures

Even though patients have the right to limit access to their private medical information, health care facilities have a duty to report certain data to governmental agencies without patient consent. These are referred to as *legally required disclosures.* Health care providers must report the following types of information to the health department:

Hello, I'd like to report a case of meningococcal meningitis.

- vital statistics, such as births and deaths

- infectious or communicable diseases, such as meningococcal meningitis, hepatitis, tuberculosis, and sexually transmitted diseases (STDs)

- any side effects caused by certain childhood vaccines

- violent injuries

While the physician is legally required to report certain information to the health department, that does not mean it's okay to share that information with someone else (such as a patient's friends or family members). For example, if a patient is diagnosed with an STD, the health department is responsible for obtaining a list of the patient's sexual partners to notify them of possible exposure to the disease. Medical office personnel, however, are required to keep the information confidential unless the patient specifies otherwise.

INITIATING TREATMENT

Initiating treatment of a new patient is the first important step when establishing a successful physician-patient relationship. As a medical assistant, you'll often be required to act as the messenger for both parties. When initiating treatment for a new patient, follow these guidelines.

1. Obtain the patient's information, including:
   - full name, with correct spelling
   - mailing address
   - day and evening phone numbers
   - reason for the office visit
   - name of the referring physician (if applicable)
   - responsible party and third party payer (insurance plan)

2. Explain the office's payment policy. Most offices require full or partial payment at the time of the first visit. Tell patients to bring all necessary insurance information to the office.

3. Make sure the patient completes proper HIPAA forms and any other medical forms. (Many medical offices mail these forms to patients and request that they bring the completed forms to their first office visit.)

4. Be sure the patient knows the location of the office and how to get there. If the patient isn't sure, offer to give her directions.

5. Ask the patient if it's permissible to leave messages on a personal or work answering machine.

6. Remind the patient of the date and time of the appointment.

7. Double-check the appointment system to make sure you've left ample room between patient visits and haven't double-booked two patients.

8. If the patient was referred by another physician, you may have to call that office and ask for copies of lab work, medical reports, and so on.

TERMINATING THE PHYSICIAN-PATIENT RELATIONSHIP

Either the patient or the physician may choose to terminate the health care relationship. A patient may terminate the relationship at any time and for any reason. The physician, however, may only terminate the physician-patient relationship due to:

- the patient's failure to pay for services
- the patient's failure to keep appointments or follow the physician's instructions
- personal reasons

Formal Written Notice

If the physician decides to end the professional relationship, she must send a letter of withdrawal to the patient that includes:

- a statement of intent to terminate the relationship
- the reason(s) for termination
- the termination date at least 30 days from the date of the letter
- a statement that medical records will be transferred to another physician at the patient's request
- a strong recommendation that the patient seek additional medical attention as needed

The termination letter must be sent by certified mail. It's also important to request a return receipt to verify that the patient was properly notified. A copy of the letter and the return receipt should then be filed in the patient's record.

When a Patient Ends the Relationship

A patient who chooses to terminate the relationship should inform the physician in writing and state the reason. You must file this letter in the patient's medical record. But whether the patient sends a formal letter or verbally requests to end the

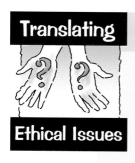

Translating

Ethical Issues

TERMINATING TREATMENT

Here are some ethical tips to remember when handling the termination of a physician-patient relationship.

- Continue to respect the patient's confidential information. Do not share this information with anyone outside the medical office, even after the patient has left the practice.
- Transfer all medical records in a timely fashion when requested.
- Make sure the patient is notified of the physician's desire to terminate the relationship. If this isn't done properly, a patient can sue for abandonment.
- Document the process appropriately. If the patient verbally asks to terminate the relationship, then the physician should send a letter to the patient documenting the conversation.

relationship, the physician should send a letter to the patient stating the following:

- The physician accepts the termination.
- The patient's medical records are available upon request.
- Medical referrals are available if needed.

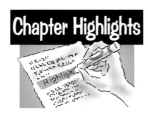

Chapter Highlights

- The components of the patient interview include obtaining a medical history, assessing signs and symptoms, gathering details about the chief complaint and present illness, and documenting the patient's history.

- Verbal communication is sending and receiving messages using words or language.

- Nonverbal communication, also known as body language, involves exchanging messages without using words. Forms of nonverbal communication include body position, facial expressions, touch, and gestures.

- Active listening is an important part of communication. You can listen actively by being engaged with what the other person is saying, supplying your full attention, and paying attention to nonverbal clues.

- When conducting patient interviews, it's helpful to use a mixture of open-ended and closed-ended questions, as well as indirect statements.

- When obtaining and recording a patient history, remember to maintain eye contact, use language the patient can understand, and listen actively to the patient's responses.

- Know the difference between sympathy and empathy. Sympathy is feeling sorry for someone, but empathy is the ability to relate to and understand another person's feelings. It's important to have empathy rather than sympathy for patients.

- Challenges to communication include language barriers, hearing impairments, cognitive impairments, and other barriers, such as indifference and sarcasm.

- Some patients may unconsciously or consciously use defense mechanisms, such as denial or rationalization. Defense mechanisms can sometimes hinder communication, so it's helpful to know how to recognize them.

- Problem-solving skills can improve your therapeutic communication with patients. With these skills, you'll be able to help the physician identify a patient's problem, develop a treatment plan, implement the plan, evaluate the results, and maintain or modify the plan.

- HIPAA, advance directives, and informed consent are examples of legal and ethical issues that affect the medical office. It's important to be aware of applicable legal and ethical issues when communicating with and about patients.

- HIPAA is the federal law that protects patient confidentiality. The guidelines set forth by HIPAA determine how private patient information must be handled in the medical office.

- HIPAA requires medical personnel to obtain patient consent before releasing medical records. Failure to follow HIPAA guidelines can lead to potentially negative consequences for the medical office.

- A physician who wishes to terminate a relationship with a patient is legally required to send formal written notice to the patient, explaining the reason for termination; transfer the patient's records to another health care provider; and recommend that the patient seek further treatment, if necessary.

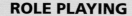

Active Learning

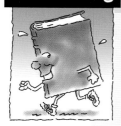

ROLE PLAYING

Divide into groups of two and come up with a brief scenario that might occur between a medical assistant and a patient. Be sure to include both verbal and nonverbal forms of communication. Then, perform your skit in front of the class. The class should then discuss each performance, identifying the verbal and nonverbal communication skills demonstrated by each group.

Observation

By yourself or with a partner, observe and list at least ten nonverbal communications that occur in the classroom. Pay attention to the following:

- facial expressions
- gestures
- body positioning

Then, explain the message of each nonverbal communication. For example, if a student scowls, you might write,

"Liz scowled when the instructor gave the class a difficult assignment. The scowl indicates that she's angry or displeased."

MEDICAL HISTORY FORM

Find a partner and complete a new patient interview, documenting your findings on the medical history form on page 129. Have one person be the interviewer and the other person be the patient and take turns playing each role. Remember that the participant answering the questions can make up the answers, instead of giving out his personal medical information to a classmate. After you've both finished, discuss what was done well during the interview and what could be improved.

Professional Medical Associates – History Form

NAME: _____ DATE OF BIRTH: _____

What is the main reason for your visit to the doctor? _____

_____

Were you referred? _____ if so, by whom? _____

PAST MEDICAL HISTORY:

Are you allergic to any medication? _____

If so, list medications: _____

List current medications, dosage, and how many times a day you take them:

Medication   **Dose**   **Times A Day**

_____

_____

Alcohol Consumption: What type? _____ Amount _____ How Often? _____

History of Alcoholism? _____

When was your last TB or Tine test? _____

Have you ever had a positive test for tuberculosis? _____

When was your last Tetanus shot? _____

List all surgeries you have had in the past:

Date   **Type of Surgery**

_____

_____

List all past hospitalizations (not involving surgeries above):

Date   **Reason For Hospital Stay**

_____

_____

List all past problems with trauma (broken bones, lacerations, etc.):

_____

REVIEW OF SYSTEMS, PAST MEDICAL PROBLEMS:
If you have been told you have any of the problems listed below, or are having any of the problems listed below, please CIRCLE:

1. GENERAL: Weight loss, weight gain, fever, chills, night sweats, hot flashes, tire easily, problems with sleep, crying spells, history of cancer.

2. SKIN: Rash, sores that won't heal, moles that are new or changing, history of skin problems.

3. HEENT: Headache, eye problems, hearing problems, sinus problems, hay fever, dizziness, hoarseness, sores in your mouth that won't heal, dental problems.

    Do you chew tobacco or dip snuff? _____

4. METABOLIC/ENDOCRINE: Thyroid problems, diabetes or sugar problems, high cholesterol.

5. RESPIRATORY: Cough, wheezing, breathing problems, history of asthma, history of lung problems.

Do you smoke cigarettes or pipe? _____

How much? _____ For how long? _____

6. BREAST (WOMEN): Breast lumps, changes in nipples, nipple discharge, breast problems, family history of breast cancer. When was your last mammogram? _____

7. CARDIOVASCULAR: Heart murmur, rheumatic fever, high blood pressure, angina, heart problems, heart attack, abnormal heart rhythm, chest pain, palpitations, leg swelling, history of phlebitis or blood clots.

8. GI: Problems with appetite, swallowing, heartburn, nausea, vomiting, pain in the abdomen, constipation, diarrhea, blood in stool, history of ulcers, liver problems, hepatitis, jaundice, pancreas problems, gallbladder problems, or colon problems.

9. REPRODUCTIVE (WOMEN): Problems with irregular menstrual cycles, abnormal vaginal bleeding or discharge, history of sexually transmitted diseases, sexual problems.

AGE OF FIRST MENSES (PERIOD) _____ AGE OF MENOPAUSE _____

LAST PAP SMEAR _____ METHOD OF CONTRACEPTION _____

Obstetric History (Women)

NUMBER OF PREGNANCIES _____ PLEASE LIST AS FOLLOWS:

Delivery Date   Pregnancy Complications   Type Delivery   Baby's Weight

_____

_____

MEN: Problems with genital discharge, history of venereal diseases, sexual problems, prostate problems.

METHOD OF CONTRACEPTION _____

10. UROLOGIC: Problems with painful urination, urinary frequency, blood in urine, weak urinary stream, history of bladder or kidney infections, or kidney stones.

11. MUSCULOSKELETAL: Arthritis, back pain, cramps in legs.

12. NEUROLOGIC: Seizures, stroke, arm or leg weakness or numbness, black-out spells, memory or thinking problems, depression, anxiety, psychiatric problems.

13. HEMATOLOGIC: Anemia, bleeding problems, enlarged lymph nodes.

HAVE YOU EVER HAD A BLOOD TRANSFUSION? _____ DATE _____

FAMILY HISTORY:

List any medical problems that run in your family and which family members have these problems.

_____

_____

SOCIAL HISTORY:

MARITAL STATUS: _____

OCCUPATION: _____

EDUCATION: _____

HOBBIES: _____

WHAT DO YOU DO FOR ENJOYMENT? _____

Chapter 5

THE CULTURALLY DIVERSE WORKPLACE

Chapter Checklist

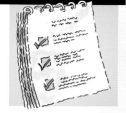

- Define culture and cultural competence

- Discuss factors that contribute to the creation of a culturally competent workplace

- List the skills necessary for communicating with a culturally diverse population

- Discuss the types of cultural differences that individuals can have with regard to their health beliefs and practices

- Employ a variety of communication skills when working with culturally diverse individuals

- Discuss some of the major health concerns of a culturally diverse population

Chapter Competencies

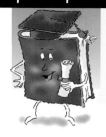

- Be attentive, listen, and learn (ABHES Competency 2.a.)

- Be impartial and show empathy when dealing with patients (ABHES Competency 2.b.)

- Recognize and respond to verbal and nonverbal communication (ABHES Competency 2.i., 2.k., and 2.l.; CAAHEP Competency 3.c.1.b. and 3.c.1.c.)

A large part of who you are is determined by the beliefs, likes, dislikes, customs, and rituals that you have. These things also affect the way you interact with others, as well as the way others interact with you. The people you work with and interact with come from various cultural backgrounds. As a medical assistant, you must be sensitive to and respectful of patients of all cultures. You can increase your sensitivity and respect by learning more about different cultures and the ways culture affects a person's life.

In this chapter, you'll examine culture as it relates to patient care. You'll look at the ways culture affects your workplace. You'll also look at the effect of culture on patient interactions. You'll see how you can use the communication tools and skills you have learned to interact effectively with people of all cultures.

Heredity, Culture, and Environment

The traits you get from your parents, the beliefs and traditions passed down from your ancestors, and everything around you affect the way you act and react. In the United States, the population is made up of people from very different backgrounds. People of different races, of different cultures, and people who speak different languages work and live side by side. As more and more people from other countries immigrate to the United States, this variation in culture will only increase. Being sensitive to and tolerant of all the different backgrounds people come from is the first step in your ability to communicate effectively with every patient you meet.

CULTURE

Your **culture** is the set of learned and shared beliefs, values, and expectations that you use in your social interactions with others. Here are some characteristics of culture:

- Your culture helps you understand what your role with others should be. It guides you to know what behavior is acceptable and unacceptable.

- You learn about your culture from your family or from others who share the same culture. Language and life experiences are the tools used to pass on the details about a culture from one person to another.

- Your social and physical environment affects how your culture is practiced. Some environments may encourage the actions of certain cultures and discourage the actions of other cultures.

- A group's culture reflects the way that group feels about itself. As a member of a certain culture, your self-image is influenced by your culture and how you feel about it.

Your culture is passed down from generation to generation.

CULTURAL COMPETENCE

Your cultural competence allows you to care effectively for patients of different cultures. **Cultural competence** is the set of beliefs, skills, and attitudes you use to interact effectively with patients of all cultures. When the cultural competence at your workplace is strong, your interactions with all patients, regardless of their cultural background, are effective. But being culturally competent is not an easy thing to accomplish. Your culture influences the way you do and say many things. It's the same with your patients. Learning to respond the right way to something a patient does or says may not happen automatically. More importantly, being able to do this all the time requires practice.

Let's look at an example. One of the first tests of your cultural competence is in the way you greet patients. And one important part of the way people greet each other is the personal space they allow between them. Personal space is the comfortable distance you keep between yourself and others. In some cultures, personal space is a very large area and physical contact in public may be unacceptable. If you interact with a patient with these cultural values, you could easily offend him by getting too close or by trying to make physical contact. But as you become culturally competent, you learn that this patient's personal space is a large area and that physical contact makes him uncomfortable.

Your cultural competence is a process that is always changing. As you interact with more and more patients, you'll learn more about different cultures. Over time and with practice, you'll discover what kinds of behavior and communication skills work best with each culture.

CRITICAL FACTORS

When you work with patients of different cultures, there are several critical factors to keep in mind. Being aware of these factors will help you know how best to communicate and interact with the patient.

Beliefs, Values, Traditions, and Practices

Make a point of getting to know each patient during your first meeting. Doing so will help you find out about the patient's cultural beliefs, values, traditions, and practices.

A good example of when this might come in handy is if you're giving dietary suggestions to a patient. In some cultures, certain foods are not permitted. Or some foods might be allowed only on certain days or at certain times of the year. Being aware of this ahead of time will help you know how to assist the patient with following the physician's instructions. As you're learning the subtle differences between cultures, do not be afraid to ask your patient a question directly. It's always acceptable to ask a question such as, "Do you have any dietary restrictions that I should be aware of?"

In some cultures, certain activities might be forbidden on certain days or at certain times of the year. If you're helping a patient work out an appointment schedule, exercise schedule, or therapy schedule, knowing which days the patient is not free is helpful.

Of course, as mentioned in other chapters, you can always ask the patient about any scheduling conflicts. Also, as you have already learned, be aware of all verbal and nonverbal clues a patient gives you. A patient may want to tell you about some culturally related issue, but may think you're not interested. Your open body stance, caring attitude, and positive body language should send the message to the patient that you want to hear what she has to say.

Culturally Defined Health-Related Needs

In some cases, the health needs of the patient, his family, or his community may be influenced by his culture. Certain procedures may not be accepted by certain cultures. Some treatment plans or parts of a treatment plan may not be allowed.

When this occurs, the physician will work with the patient to explore other options. Giving the patient as many choices as possible allows the patient to take responsibility for his own health care. By providing options, the health care team shows that it's open to working with the patient to meet her needs.

Culturally Based Belief Systems

Some cultures have strong beliefs about the cause of illness and disease or about the nature of health and healing. A patient may wish to share with you his ideas about what caused his ulcer, or about why his headache went away. As always, listen actively and sincerely. Always remember your goal as a medical assistant—to help meet the health care needs of the patient.

Culturally Based Attitudes

Some patients may have preferences about whether or not they seek help from health care providers. Some patients may have a preference about whether a male or female helps them with their health care needs. Be prepared to resolve these culturally based attitudes as best as you can.

In some cultures, females are not allowed to hold positions of importance. If you're a female and a patient would rather see a male medical assistant, do not take it personally. Respect the patient's cultural beliefs by doing what you can to honor the patient's request.

BUILDING A CULTURALLY COMPETENT WORKPLACE

The patients you interact with will likely be made up of people from many other cultures. Your goal as a medical assistant is to develop the knowledge and practice the skills necessary to provide culturally competent care to all patients.

From the moment a patient enters the medical office, she must feel welcomed. The attitudes of all who work in the office should be positive. Read through the following ways that you can help create a more culturally competent workplace.

Value Diversity

You have your own beliefs about illness and health. But your beliefs are probably not the same as those of others. The attitudes and beliefs people have about their health are highly influenced by their culture. There are many different cultures in the United States. This variety is referred to as **diversity.** Because there is great cultural diversity in the United States, there is also great diversity of beliefs and attitudes about health and illness.

Be sure to celebrate and value the diversity reflected in your patients. Let all patients know that you respect their cultural beliefs and attitudes by communicating with them sincerely and effectively.

Assess Your Own Cultural Beliefs

In order for you to accept the diversity in cultural beliefs about health, it's important for you to first know what your own beliefs are. This might be difficult at first. After all, the culture you grow up in is what is "real" for you. It's not always easy to think about or question the ideas you were raised with. What are your own beliefs about health and illness? Do you have any time-honored remedies that you wouldn't be able to locate in a medical textbook? Are there things you do at home for a cold or fever that your grandmother used to do? Did you ever have a high fever as a child and have someone in your family say, "Starve a cold; feed a fever!" to get you to eat something? Maybe some of these ideas are part of your culture, rather than your medical training.

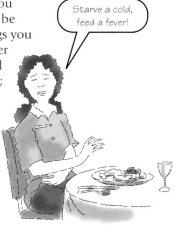

Starve a cold, feed a fever!

We all have our own beliefs about health and illness.

Appreciate Differences Between Cultures

Cultures differ in ways other than attitudes about health and illness. People from different cultures may wear different kinds of clothes, they may speak a different language, they may eat different foods, and they may think very differently about certain topics. This is a good thing! Imagine a world in which everyone ate, dressed, thought, and talked the same. How boring!

Accepting the differences between cultures allows you to see and hear about other ways of life. You may sometimes disagree with what somebody else thinks about something. But appreciating that the differences exist is a key part of your role as a medical assistant.

Find Out About Other Cultures

Suppose you're treating a young woman who has just emigrated here from Croatia in Eastern Europe. She is quiet and reserved and does not say much since she is still learning how to speak English. To help her feel more comfortable, find out more about her country. Take time to research her culture. Look on the Internet or go to the local library to see what information you can find about Croatia and its culture.

Taking time to find out about other cultures shows your sincere interest in your patients. In the course of your research, you'll learn not only about other cultures, but you might find that you better understand your own culture, too.

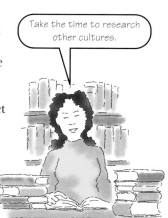

Take the time to research other cultures.

Adapt to Another's Cultural Beliefs and Practices

Whenever possible, do what you can to adapt to a patient's cultural beliefs and practices. For example, suppose a patient tells you that she can't make her next appointment because she will be observing a traditional holiday. Honor your

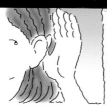

Listen to This | CULTURAL COMPETENCE CHECKLIST

When interacting with patients of different cultures, keep this cultural competence checklist in mind. Review each of the factors listed below to see how culturally competent your patient interactions are.

Am I being sensitive to the patient's:

- beliefs, values, traditions, and practices
- culturally defined health-related needs
- culturally based beliefs
- culturally based attitudes

patient's traditions by doing what you can to reschedule her appointment to one she can make. Respecting the beliefs and practices of your patients will help build a more solid relationship.

Communicating with a Culturally Diverse Population

One of your primary goals as a medical assistant is to communicate effectively with your patients. But what if the patient speaks a language other than the one you use? Being able to communicate with patients whose language is not your own is a challenge. But there are ways you can break through the language barrier and still communicate effectively.

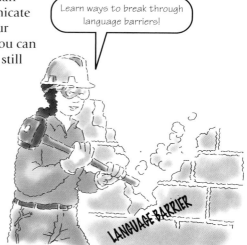

Learn ways to break through language barriers!

LINGUISTIC COMPETENCE

As you know, you and your coworkers must be able to communicate effectively with all patients. This includes those who speak different languages. The ability to do this in your work environment is called **linguistic competence**. You and your coworkers must communicate in a way that patients of all cultures can understand. To build up your office's linguistic competence, keep these points in mind:

Listen

Listen to the patient's verbal and nonverbal communication. What do his gestures say to you about how he feels? What does the patient think is the problem?

Offer Feedback

Once you have listened to all the patient has to say, offer feedback. Confirm with the patient as best you can that you understand what he is trying to tell you. Let the patient know you appreciate and care about his well-being. Allow the patient to share more if he would like to do so.

Ask for Clarification

Do not hesitate to ask for clarification. If you do not understand something the patient has said, ask him to explain. The act of making something clearer and easier to understand is called **clarification**. Asking for clarification helps strengthen the communication between you and the patient. And when you ask for clarification, it sends a message to the patient that he can feel free to ask you for clarification as well.

Assess

Assess the impact of cultural differences on whatever treatment options a patient has been given. If you see a conflict between a prescribed treatment option and the patient's cultural practices, you may need to notify the physician. It's important to know enough about a patient's cultural background to know if a treatment option is acceptable or not.

The Cultural Guidebook

Your culture is like a guidebook that you follow throughout your life. It tells you which kinds of behavior are okay and which are not. It gives you certain beliefs, rules, and customs that become part of your everyday life. What's more, because everyone with the same culture as you uses the same "guidebook," you and the other members of your culture share a common ground from which you make important life decisions. In this way, the cultural guidebook is what connects people from the same culture. If you know nothing about another person's culture (in other words, you're not familiar with another

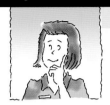

Say it Isn't So

HOW CAN YOU COMMUNICATE WITH PATIENTS WHO DO NOT SPEAK ENGLISH?

What are some ways to communicate with Spanish-speaking patients?

A couple is expecting their first baby. Both the mother and father speak only Spanish. They are concerned about the pregnancy, labor, and delivery. They would like to take classes to help them prepare. You have a limited Spanish vocabulary, as do a few of your coworkers. Should you try to communicate with the couple using only the few Spanish phrases you know?

This is a perfect example for which printed resources can help. Many brochures and pamphlets are printed in other languages, especially Spanish. Make sure your office has a supply of frequently requested brochures. Popular topics include:

- pregnancy
- drug abuse
- SIDS
- aging
- nutrition
- exercise

Also, keep a list of phone numbers for community resources that are available for Spanish-speaking members of the community. It's possible that pregnancy classes are offered in Spanish. Explore videos and DVDs as well. Many are available in multiple languages, or with language subtitles.

person's guidebook), your interactions with that person might be confusing.

For example, let's say you're about to meet, for the first time, a patient who grew up in Culture X. One of the customs in the "Culture X Guidebook" is that instead of shaking hands when they meet, members of Culture X grasp each others' shoulders with their right hands. Since childhood, people from Culture X are taught this custom. Everyone from Culture X greets each other this way. But you know nothing about Culture X. Therefore you have no way of knowing about this custom. So when you first meet the patient from Culture X, he greets you with a hearty grasp of your shoulder. You would probably be a little confused! In a situation such as this, try to recognize the patient's nonverbal cues. Is he smiling while grasping your shoulder? If so, his gesture probably means the same thing as a handshake does in your culture.

> A warm greeting means the same thing in every culture, even if the action is a little bit different.

CULTURAL DIFFERENCES AND THE MEDICAL ASSISTANT

As a medical assistant, one of your first goals is to know how patients' cultural backgrounds might affect your interactions with them. Let patients know that you welcome the chance to learn about their culture. Do not be afraid to ask questions. The more you know about a patient's culture, the easier it will be for you to help him with his health plan.

Health Beliefs

Many cultures have specific beliefs, customs, and practices about health and illness. You can ask the patient directly what these are. You can also research them on your own. Some areas related to health beliefs are discussed below.

Food and Diet

People of different cultures may use certain foods as staples in their everyday diets. For example, rice and vegetables are staples of the Asian diet. Pasta is a staple of the Italian diet. The Hispanic diet uses a lot of tortillas. In some cultures, people might eat their largest meal late at night, or they might eat many small meals throughout the day. Some cultures might recommend fasting for one or more days on a regular basis. In any case, find out what the cultural rules for food and diet are for your patients.

Medication

A patient might choose to avoid using some or all medications recommended to her. In some cultures, nonmedication treatments for some illnesses are preferred. It is very important that you remain open-minded with all patients. If a patient shares with you that he prefers not taking a prescribed medication, pass this information on to the physician. Remember that your goal is to work with each patient to help him meet his health

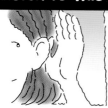

Listen to This   CULTURAL DIFFERENCES IN NUTRITION

To test your cultural awareness about diet and nutrition, ask yourself the following questions:

1. Which foods are considered edible and which are not?
   - In France, corn is considered animal feed, whereas corn is a commonly eaten vegetable in the United States.
   - Religious beliefs prohibit some Jewish, Muslim, and Seventh-Day Adventist patients from eating pork.
   - Patients who follow a vegetarian diet do not eat pork, beef, or chicken.

2. What times and types of food are considered meals?
   - Anglo-Americans typically eat three meals a day, with foods such as bacon and eggs or cereal for breakfast, sandwiches and soup for lunch, and meat with potatoes and vegetables for dinner.
   - Vietnamese people may eat soup for every meal.
   - Beans are a staple for meals among Mexican people.
   - People from Middle Eastern countries often eat cheese and olives for breakfast.
   - Native American and Latin American people usually eat two meals a day.
   - Rural southern African Americans may eat large amounts of food on weekends and less food at meals during the week.
   - Holy days and religious holidays influence food choices for almost all cultures.

care needs. You might disagree with the patient's decision to refuse prescription medication, but in this instance, your professional obligation to the patient must come before your personal beliefs about what is right. If you know the patient is not willing to follow a particular plan, your duty is to inform the physician so that the physician can consider alternate therapies for the patient.

Other Forms of Care

Many cultures use various types of health care. Faith healers, acupuncture, acupressure, herbs, voodoo, and skilled elders may be part of a patient's health care plan.

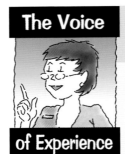

The Voice of Experience

WORKING WITH PATIENTS WHO WILL NOT TAKE MEDICATION

Q: *How do I work with a patient whose religious beliefs prevent her from taking pain medication?*

A: When pain medication has been prescribed to a patient, the patient has the choice of taking the medication or not. If a patient tells you that she prefers not taking pain medication, you must respect the patient's decision. You might ask the patient what her plan is for dealing with pain. Some people might prefer to use meridian therapy, acupressure, acupuncture, acumassage, or meditation to help them manage their pain. Some might use pain medication only as a last resort.

Above all, listen to the patient's views regarding health and illness. Learn what you can about the patient's opinions and beliefs. You'll be able to better assist the patient if you first understand how she approaches her own health care.

Some patients might believe strongly in a holistic approach to health. **Holistic** means that the whole body—spiritual, physical, emotional, and psychological—is treated. For example, a patient with arthritis will treat not only the arthritis itself (the physical part of the disease process), but may also meditate to help heal the spiritual, emotional, and psychological parts of her being. Holistic medicine treats not just the part of the body that is ill or injured. It treats the body as a whole.

The Body

People have different levels of understanding about the way the body works. Some patients may have no understanding at all about how or why their body is ill or how it heals. On the other hand, other patients may have a high level of understanding of how their body functions.

Patients with little or no knowledge will not understand technical details about their health treatment. Patients with a lot of knowledge will often *want* to know the details of their health treatment. It is very important for you to be aware of the level of knowledge that your patients have and want. If a patient tells you that she wants to know more details about her treatment, be sure to let the physician know.

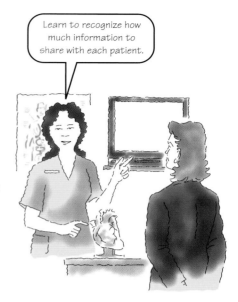

Learn to recognize how much information to share with each patient.

Folk Healers

As you have already learned, a patient's religious beliefs are part of her cultural guidebook. As a result, many religious beliefs affect a patient's response to illness, disease, and death. In some cultures, a folk healer is a person thought to have a special gift for making others well. As with the other health beliefs discussed here, be aware that these are all part of the way a patient approaches her health treatment plan. It's your job as a medical assistant to take all of these beliefs into consideration when helping your patients.

Traditions and Rituals

A patient's culture may have certain traditions or rituals that are practiced either individually or as a group. Some cultures may have certain practices, holidays, and celebrations related to childbirth, puberty, marriage, or death. A patient might share information about these traditions or rituals with you. You may even be invited to participate. Keep an open mind and a willing spirit if this happens. Such sharing turns opportunities like these into enriching cultural experiences for everyone.

Courtesies and Customs

Every culture has its own set of everyday courtesies and customs. Some of these are quite different from your own. Some are just a little bit different. For example, what people do and say when they greet each other can vary a lot from culture to culture. Did you know that in some South Asian cultures, being late is considered a sign of respect? In some cultures, people greet each other using a double handshake, or by clapping, or by squeezing each other's fingers. What is said during a greeting differs, too. Instead of "How are you?" other cultures greet each other with phrases that mean "Speak!" "Have you eaten?" or "On you no evil."

Be open to all customs and courtesies of other cultures. Never assume that the traditions of your culture are known or accepted by everyone. Always be aware of any nonverbal clues that tell you when a patient is uncomfortable about something that has been done or said.

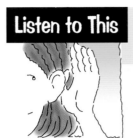

Listen to This

APPLYING CROSS-CULTURAL UNDERSTANDING TO HEALTH CARE

One of the goals of cultural knowledge and awareness is improving cross-cultural understanding and communication. Being familiar with cultural characteristics, history, values, and belief systems increases our cultural knowledge without stereotyping individuals of a particular culture. When we are culturally sensitive, we know that similarities and differences exist within each culture.

The table below summarizes various practices, beliefs, and health problems that may be common to certain cultural groups. Considering these factors (and being aware that they may not apply to *all* members of a particular cultural group) is an important part of providing culturally competent health care.

Cultural Factors That Affect Health Care	
Cultural Group	**Cultural Factors**
Caucasian	Family: • Nuclear family is highly valued. • Elderly family members may live in a nursing home when they can no longer care for themselves. Folk and traditional health care: • self-diagnosis of illness • use of over-the-counter drugs (especially vitamins and pain relievers) • dieting (especially fad diets) • extensive use of exercise and exercise facilities Values and beliefs: • youth valued over age • cleanliness • orderliness • attractiveness • individualism • achievement • punctuality Common health problems: • cardiovascular diseases • gastrointestinal diseases • some forms of cancer • motor vehicle accidents • suicides • mental illness • substance abuse

Cultural Group	Cultural Factors
African American	Family: • close and supportive extended family relationships • strong kinship ties with nonblood relatives from church or organizational and social groups • importance of family unity, loyalty, and cooperation • usually matriarchal Folk and traditional health care varies extensively and may or may not include: • spiritualists • herb/root doctors • conjurers • skilled elder family members • voodoo • faith healing Values and beliefs: • present oriented • high respect for members of the African-American clergy • frequently highly religious Common health problems: • hypertension • sickle cell anemia • skin disorders, such as inflammation of hair follicles, various types of dermatitis, and excessive growth of scar tissue (keloids) • lactose enzyme deficiency, resulting in poor tolerance of milk products • higher rate of tuberculosis • diabetes mellitus • higher infant mortality rate than in the white population
Asian	Family: • Welfare of the family is valued above the person. • Extended families are common. • A person's lineage (ancestral line) is respected. • Sharing among family members is expected. Folk and traditional health care: • Theoretical basis is in Taoism, which seeks balance in all things. • Good health is achieved through the proper balance of yin (feminine, negative, dark, cold) and yang (masculine, positive, light, warm). • An imbalance in energy is caused by an improper diet or strong emotions.

(continued)

Cultural Factors That Affect Health Care (*Continued*)

Cultural Group	Cultural Factors

- Diseases and foods are classified as hot or cold, and a proper balance between them will promote wellness (for example, treat a cold disease with hot foods).
- Many Asian health care systems use herbs, diet, and the application of hot or cold therapy. Also, many Asians believe that there are points on the body that are located on the meridians or energy pathways. If the energy flow is out of balance, treatment (such as acu-massage, acupressure, or acupuncture) may be necessary to restore the energy equilibrium.

Values and beliefs:
- strong sense of self-respect and self-control
- high respect for age
- respect for authority
- respect for hard work
- praise of self or others considered poor manners
- strong emphasis on harmony and the avoidance of conflict

Common health problems:
- tuberculosis
- communicable diseases
- malnutrition
- suicide
- various forms of mental illness
- lactose enzyme deficiency

Hispanic

Family:
- Familial role is important.
- *Compadrazgo* is the term used to describe the special bond between a child's parents and his godparents.
- Family is the primary unit of society.

Folk and traditional health care:
- *Curanderas* or *curanderos* are frequently folk healers who base treatments on the belief that the basic functions of the body are controlled by four body fluids or "humors." These four body fluids include blood (hot and wet), yellow bile (hot and dry), black bile (cold and dry), and phlegm (cold and wet).
- The secret of good health is to balance hot and cold within the body. Therefore, most foods, beverages, herbs, and medications are classified as hot (*caliente*) or cold (*fresco, frio*). For example, a cold disease will be cured with a hot treatment.

Cultural Group	Cultural Factors
	Values and beliefs:
	• Respect is given according to age (older) and gender (male).
	• Roman Catholic Church may be very influential.
	• God gives health and allows illness for a reason. Therefore, many perceive illness as a punishment from God. An illness of this type can be cured through atonement and forgiveness.
	Common health problems:
	• diabetes mellitus and its complications
	• poverty and resultant problems, such as poor nutrition, inadequate medical care, poor prenatal care
	• lactose enzyme deficiency
Puerto Rican	Family:
	• *compadrazgo*—same as in Hispanic culture
	Folk and traditional health care practices are similar to those of other Spanish-speaking cultures.
	Values and beliefs:
	• High value is placed on safeguarding against group pressure to violate a person's integrity. For example, it may be difficult for a person who holds this belief to accept teamwork.
	• People should remain close-mouthed about personal and family affairs (a belief that may make psychotherapy difficult).
	• Proper consideration should be given to cultural rituals such as shaking hands and standing up to greet and say good-bye to people.
	• Time is a relative phenomenon; little attention is given to the exact time of day.
	• *Ataques,* which is characterized by hyperkinetic seizure activity, is a culturally acceptable reaction to situations of extreme stress.
	Common health problems:
	• parasitic diseases, such as dysentery, malaria, filariasis, and hookworms
	• lactose enzyme deficiency
Native American	Family:
	• Families are large and extended.
	• Grandparents are official and symbolic leaders and decision makers.
	• A child's namesake may become the same as another parent to the child.
	Folk and traditional health care:
	• Medicine men (*shamans*) are widely used.
	• Herbs, psychological treatments, ceremonies, fasting, meditation, heat, and massages are heavily used.

(*continued*)

Cultural Factors That Affect Health Care (*Continued*)

Cultural Group	Cultural Factors

Values and beliefs:
- Beliefs are present oriented. Children are taught to live in the present and not to be concerned about the future. This time consciousness emphasizes finishing current business before doing something else.
- There is a high respect for age.
- Great value is placed on working together and sharing resources.
- Failure to achieve a personal goal is frequently believed to be the result of competition.
- High respect is given to a person who gives to others. The accumulation of money and goods is often frowned upon.
- Some Native Americans practice the Peyotist religion, in which the consumption of peyote, an intoxicating drug derived from mescal cacti, is part of the service. Peyote is legal if used for this purpose. It's classified as a hallucinogenic drug.

NOTE: Each tribe's beliefs and practices vary to some degree.

Common health problems:
- alcoholism
- suicide
- tuberculosis
- malnutrition
- communicable diseases
- higher maternal and infant mortality rates than in other populations
- diabetes mellitus
- hypertension
- gallbladder disease

Hawaiian

Family:
- *Ohana,* or extended families, are jointly involved in childrearing.
- Hierarchy of familial structure is important; each gender and age has specific duties.
- Closely knit families may live in small, isolated communities.

Folk and traditional health care:
- *Kahuna la'au lapa'nu* is the ancient Hawaiian medical practitioner.
- A patient's illness is viewed as part of the whole.
- Relationships between the physical, psychological, and spiritual are important.
- The use of preventive medicine is emphasized.
- More than 300 medicinal plants and minerals are used in treatment.

Cultural Group	Cultural Factors

Values and beliefs:
- *aloha*—a deep love, respect, and affection between people and the land
- respect given to people and the land
- lifestyle more revered than compliance with health care issues
- present oriented
- death seen as part of life and not feared

Common health problems:
- diabetes mellitus and its complications
- hypertension (unknown cause; perhaps related to diet)
- gout (perhaps related to diet)
- respiratory disorders, such as asthma, allergies, and tuberculosis
- bacterial or fungal skin disorders and skin cancer

(Adapted with permission from Taylor C, Lillis C, LeMone P. *Fundamentals of Nursing: The Art and Science of Nursing Care,* 5th ed. Philadelphia: Lippincott Williams & Wilkins, 2005.)

Family Interactions

The ways that families deal with health care issues can differ greatly from culture to culture. For instance, in some families, it may be unacceptable to share any private health information at all with non-family members, including you and any other health care provider.

In some families, there may be one person who makes all the health-related decisions for everyone else. If this is the case, a patient might need approval from this family member before any part of a treatment plan can begin. However, a situation such as this brings up the question of whether you should or should not share an adult patient's private health information with another person, even if that person is the patient's spouse or parent. Before you address the cultural rules for sharing a patient's information, you must first consider the patient's HIPAA privacy rights. After you have obtained the patient's consent to share his private health information with specific people, you may then be faced with the challenge of how to balance respect for cultural differences with your goal of providing the best care for the patient.

As you have learned, culture affects how patients interact with you. As a medical assistant, you must be aware of cultural differences between you and your patients so that you can interact with them as effectively as possible. You must also have an idea about how culture changes the way a family interacts with you. In some cultures, the family is very involved in the health of all its members. It's up to you to learn how you can work with the traditions of a family so that the needs of the patient can be met.

Family Roles and Decision Making

You may find that in some families, there is one person who makes most of the important decisions. This person might be the father, mother, or a grandparent. If you see that a patient's family works this way, find out which family member is considered the decision maker. Be sure to involve this person as much as possible.

Gender, Age, and Family Position

In many cultures, older family members are considered the wisest. In some cultures, only the oldest male is allowed to make important decisions. In other cultures, it's the oldest female.

The roles of each child might be different, too. The oldest child may be allowed to make certain health-related decisions, but the youngest child may not be allowed to make any. As with the other issues discussed in this chapter, find out what the customs and rules are in the patient's family.

Grief and Bereavement

The loss of a family member or friend brings sadness and grief. You show your grief in your own way. Families show their grief in their own way. Culture affects the ways that individuals and families grieve. Some people may be very open about their grief. Others may prefer to grieve in private.

Know how you feel about dying and death. Understanding your own feelings about death will help you better understand the feelings of your patient. This will help you meet the needs of your patient and of your patient's family if they are ever faced with a personal loss.

IMPACT ON PATIENT INTERACTIONS

Remember that your goal as a medical assistant is to help meet a patient's health needs. But you may find that cultural differences get in the way of your being able to reach that goal. Recognizing these conflicts early in your patient interaction will help you figure out how best to solve them. A cultural conflict may not appear until you have known a patient for a while. Or there may be no conflicts at all.

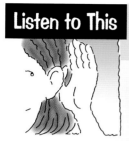

Listen to This

PREPARING YOURSELF FOR DEATH AND DYING

Your personal feelings about death and dying are the basis for the way you're able to help patients deal with these same issues. The following are some questions you should ask yourself about how you feel about death and dying.

What would I want in the room?

- What location would I choose for my own death? Would I prefer to be at home or in a hospital?

- If I could, what cause of death would I choose? Why?

- Whom would I want to have present at my death? What kinds of objects, music, lighting, and furniture would I want in the room?

- What fears do I have about death? Why do I have these fears?

- How do I think my patients would answer these questions?

Examine your own feelings about death and dying as a way to connect with your patients.

Here are some ways that you can avoid culture-related conflict with your patients' care.

Evaluate the Conflict

Your first meeting with a patient should give you an idea about whether cultural conflicts might exist. If you suspect they might, consider which of your patient's beliefs could interfere with his health care. Research the patient's culture, beliefs, and customs. Discuss your concerns with the physician. Speak with the patient as you start to feel more comfortable talking about these issues. Involving the patient is an important step in these situations. However, be careful to consider whether doing so goes against what the patient's family feels is acceptable.

Work Out a Plan

Of course whenever possible, you want to avoid conflicts between a certain health care plan and a patient's lifestyle or beliefs. In the case of a conflict, always work with the physician to explore other options. If necessary, involve the family in working out an acceptable plan.

Be an Educator

Remember that patients' knowledge and understanding about health and medical treatments may vary greatly. Whenever necessary, try to educate patients who might have no knowledge or incorrect knowledge about their health. Keep in mind that some cultures may pass down from generation to generation incorrect or inaccurate explanations for certain health conditions.

Are You Culturally Competent?

How can you be sure if you're culturally competent? What about your workplace? How can you tell if your office is set up to meet the needs of patients of all cultures? The cultural competence of you and your coworkers shows in many ways.

Becoming culturally competent takes work, but the rewards are more than worth it!

VALUES AND ATTITUDES

Your values and attitudes toward your patients come through in the way you interact with them. Understanding and accepting any differences between your own set of values and those of your patients is the first step toward cultural competence. You can work to take this first step yourself, or, if you're already well on your way to being culturally competent, you can help your coworkers take this important first step.

Policies and Procedures

The medical office should represent cultural competence in all its policies and procedures. The ways you and your coworkers respond to culturally sensitive issues must be consistent. In other words, your approach to a culturally sensitive issue must be the same as that of your coworkers. This kind of consistency strengthens cultural competence.

For example, let's say the physician has prescribed a certain medication to a patient. The patient tells you that he would like to try his family's herbal remedy before taking the prescribed medicine. Your response to this patient's choice should be the same as the way a coworker would respond. And if you're in doubt about how to respond, you should be able to look up your medical office's policies for just such a situation. If there is no policy in place, you might want to notify the physician or office manager.

No Bias, No Judgment

As you have read, the policies and procedures practiced by you and your coworkers must be consistent. However, consistency is only half the battle. Your medical office's policies and procedures must also be free of any bias or judgment.

Let's go back to the example of a patient who wants to try an herbal remedy rather than traditional prescription medication. No matter how you feel about this choice, your response to this patient must be free of any judgmental words or phrases. However, you should inform the physician of the patient's herbal remedy plan and document it in the patient's chart. The physician can then decide the best course of action for this patient.

PHYSICAL ENVIRONMENT, MATERIALS, AND RESOURCES

Before a patient interacts with you, he interacts with your office. In some cases, a patient may spend more time in the waiting room than in the examination room. How do you think patients feel when they walk into your office? Do they feel welcomed? Is the atmosphere warm and friendly? Setting up an environment in which all patients feel comfortable is the first step in creating a positive experience for everyone.

Culturally Diverse Atmosphere

Know your patients. This is your first step to creating an atmosphere in your office that is comfortable for all patients. Provide pamphlets, brochures, magazines, videos, and other materials in multiple languages.

Nonverbal Communication Tools

The things that a patient looks at in the office should be pleasing and positive. Make sure any art or photographs on the walls are respectful. All slogans, pictures, or posters should present a positive message. Some offices feature the art or photography of a different local artist every month or so. This is a great artistic way to increase the cultural competence of your workplace.

Literacy Level

You probably have many brochures and informational materials available to patients. Make sure that any written materials your office provides are available at all reading levels. Remember that

Send and Receive

COMMUNICATING WITHOUT BIAS OR JUDGMENT

Here is an example of an ineffective and effective dialogue between a medical assistant and the patient who wants to use an herbal remedy before trying the medication prescribed by the physician.

Ineffective:

- "Here is your prescription, Mr. Diaz. Remember, the physician directed you to take two tablets every 12 hours." You give Mr. Diaz the prescription.

- Mr. Diaz pauses while looking at the prescription, and then says, "I think I'd like to try a different approach first. There is an herbal tea that my grandmother makes. People in my family use it often for this kind of ailment."

- You roll your eyes and snicker as you say, "Well, sure, I guess if you really want to. When your tea doesn't work, give us a call."

You must treat a patient's cultural preferences with respect. Let the patient know that you respect his approach and attitude. You do this with your verbal and nonverbal communication skills.

Effective:

- "Here is your prescription, Mr. Diaz. Remember, the physician directed you to take two tablets every 12 hours. Do you have any questions or concerns?"

- Mr. Diaz pauses while looking at the prescription, and then says, "I think I'd like to try a different approach first. There is an herbal tea that my grandmother makes. People in my family use it often for this kind of ailment."

- You smile and say, "Of course. I'll let the physician know. He may call you if he has a concern about the tea. Do you happen to know what the herbs are? I'd like to include this information in your medical chart."

Many cultures have different approaches to illness. A patient may prefer to try a treatment other than the one a physician prescribes. The most important part of this scenario is that you listen to what the patient wants to do and share that information with the physician. In this way, you show respect for the patient and his cultural preferences, and you also learn more about the alternate approach. The more you know, the better able you'll be to inform the physician of the patient's intent. If the physician sees a potential problem, he can speak with the patient directly.

children like to learn about health and their bodies, too. Be sure to provide materials that they can look at by themselves or with others.

COMMUNICATION STYLES

You'll probably see patients who speak a language that is different from yours. You might not know any language other than your own. But that does not mean you can't learn enough of another language to be able to communicate at least a little. You can prepare ahead of time for a patient who speaks Spanish or French or Swahili by learning a common greeting in her native language and a bit about her culture.

> Learn a few key phrases in a patient's own language.

Learning Key Phrases

You do not have time to become fluent in the language of every patient you see. But it can be very helpful to learn at least a few key phrases, such as simple questions that will give you more information about the patient's medical complaints. Your interactions with a patient are usually limited to greetings and health topics. Learning how to say simple things like "Hello," "How are you feeling?", "Good-bye," and "Where does it hurt?" can be very useful. So for example, if you have a patient who speaks Swahili and only a little English, learn some Swahili words before the patient's next visit.

Bilingual Staff or Interpreters

Learning a few things to say to patients who speak a different language is helpful. But having a bilingual person in your office is an even bigger help. A person who is **bilingual** can speak and understand two languages. If you're seeing a patient who understands nothing you say, it's very helpful to have somebody in your office who speaks that patient's language and can serve as an interpreter. This will save much time and frustration for both you and the patient.

Writing in the Patient's First Language

A patient receives many kinds of written information from you and from the physician. A patient who has trouble speaking English probably has trouble reading it, too. Whenever possible, write down appointment reminders, medication instructions, and other health information in the patient's first language. This is another way you help guarantee the patient's understanding.

Accessing Community Resources

Do not forget that your community is a great place to get extra support and information. You can contact advocacy groups, alliances, religious organizations, and other support groups. These groups are usually happy to do what they can to strengthen the cultural competence of your workplace. Have their business cards and brochures handy so that you can give them to patients when needed.

Providing Culturally Competent Care

The United States includes a mixture of cultures and races. It makes sense to assume that, as a medical assistant, you'll interact with coworkers and patients of many different cultures and races. Knowing this, it therefore makes sense to make yourself and your workplace as culturally competent as possible. As discussed earlier, one way you do this is by making sure policies are in place to help you and your coworkers deal effectively with any cultural issues that might come up. Here are some other ways to help build cultural competence.

AVOID CULTURAL BIAS AND STEREOTYPING

In a work environment that is not culturally competent, two things are likely to happen—cultural bias and stereotyping. **Bias** happens when your personal opinion affects the way you treat another person. Let's say you do not like the color blue. In fact, you really dislike the color blue and anything that is blue. Now let's say you meet a patient who is dressed all in blue. You might have a tendency to be biased against the patient because she is dressed in blue. You may not be as friendly or courteous to her. You may not explain information as thoroughly. Your body language may not be as open as it should be.

Cultural bias is a bias against a certain culture. Instead of being biased against people who wear the color blue, a cultural bias is directed at the people of a certain culture.

Stereotyping means having an opinion of a certain culture, race, religion, age group, or other group that is based on something negative or oversimplified. Some stereotypes you may have already come across include the beliefs that men never cry, older adults are grumpy, or that all medical assistants are female. While it may be true that some men never cry, it's a stereotype to assume that all men never cry, or that only women cry.

As you can probably guess, biases and stereotyping make it difficult to establish positive relationships between people. As a medical assistant, any bias or stereotyping you show toward coworkers or patients will get in the way of effective interactions and positive communications.

ALL CULTURES ARE IMPORTANT

It's possible that your culture is different from the majority of your patients. Or it could be that the culture of the community in which you work is different from yours. It's important to understand the needs and cultural background of the community where you work. The majority of the people in an office or community might follow one culture. But this does not mean that the culture of another person is less important.

INTERVENE WHEN OTHERS ARE CULTURALLY INSENSITIVE

What should you do if you observe others being culturally insensitive? If this happens, you should be quick to step in and intervene.

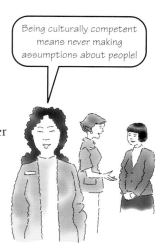

Being culturally competent means never making assumptions about people!

For example, let's say one of your coworkers is about to interview a new patient, Mr. Ling. On her way to meeting Mr. Ling in the waiting room, the coworker comments to you, "I sure hope I do not need an interpreter for this guy." Your coworker is making an assumption that just because the patient's name is Ling, he will speak English poorly or not at all. You could remind your coworker that many people who are born and raised in this country have foreign last names. Point out that Mr. Ling might know *only* English and not a word of any other language!

PROVIDING SERVICES

As you begin to learn about the many different cultures your medical office serves, you can begin to develop routines for effectively serving each culture. For example, suppose you're aware that the people in your community are predominantly members of a certain cultural group. You know that members of this cultural group have one of the highest incidences of hypertension relative to other cultural groups in your area. You should be aware that the treatment and prevention of hypertension will be an issue of common concern among your patients. Your office should have relevant education pamphlets and brochures available. You should also have a list of community resources for your patients to access. You may also want to participate in projects in schools and in your community that are geared toward hypertension education and disease prevention.

COMMUNICATION TIPS

This and other chapters have discussed communication skills and strategies. No matter what the age, race, religion, or culture of a patient, the way you communicate with that patient must be positive and effective. Communicating with patients who do not speak English requires a slightly different approach. Here are some tips to keep in mind:

- Speak slowly, not loudly. Raising your voice will not help patients understand you any better.
- Face the patient. Keep good eye contact when speaking to the patient, but do not expect the patient to do the same. In some cultures, downcast eyes are a sign of respect.
- Use short, simple sentences. The patient may understand a little bit of English, so using simple questions that require simple answers will help.
- Use gestures, pictures, and facial expressions. There are many gestures and facial expressions that all people understand. An open palm can be used to say, "Stop." You can pantomime drinking a glass of water to show a patient that a medication should be taken with liquids.
- Observe body language carefully. Watch the patient for feedback about his understanding. His facial expression might let you know that he does not understand what you just said.
- Be open-minded when a patient uses gestures or facial expressions with which you're unfamiliar.
- Avoid difficult and uncommon words. A patient who understands only a little bit of English will be confused if you use long or technical words. Keep the language simple.
- Avoid idiomatic expressions. Stay away from phrases or sayings that a patient who is not fluent in English

will not understand. Examples of idiomatic expressions include, "You'll sleep like a log" and "Do not add fuel to the fire."

- Rephrase and summarize often. If you see that the patient is confused or isn't responding to what you've said, repeat yourself. If you've had to give the patient a lot of information, take some time to summarize.

- Ask open questions. Especially with patients who speak little English, it can be tempting to ask a series of "yes" or "no" questions. But these questions limit the information a patient can give you. It's better to take the time to ask open questions and work with the patient to understand his answers.

- Check your understanding of the patient by providing feedback. Let the patient know that you understand what he has said to you. Give the patient as much verbal and nonverbal feedback as you can.

MAJOR HEALTH CONCERNS FOR OUR CULTURALLY DIVERSE POPULATION

In a country with so many different cultures, you should be aware of some special health concerns that exist. In preparing to be culturally competent, you should expect to deal with certain health issues connected to geography, poverty, and heredity.

Some health issues are related to the plants that live in an area.

Where You Are Matters

Some health issues are a result of where people live. Many people live in areas that are far from a town or city. A rural setting makes it difficult for patients to get proper health care when they need it. People who live in areas that are sunny and hot most of the year may have more health issues connected to sunstroke and skin cancer. The types of plants that grow in an area may also result in certain health issues. Coming in contact with poison oak, poison ivy, or stinging nettles, and eating poisonous berries are some examples.

Money Matters

Poverty is a serious problem in this country. Children, older adults, and single-parent families are especially at risk when they are living in conditions of poverty. For example, many people who are poor live on a fixed income, which means they often have no extra money to pay for prescriptions or office visits if a medical condition occurs. A person in this situation may choose to "wait it out" rather than seek medical care. As a result, the person may become much sicker and require emergency hospital care. There are no easy solutions to the problem of poverty.

In your role as a medical assistant, you need to begin to look for signs of poverty, such as medical conditions that go untreated or prescriptions that are not filled. If you suspect a patient in your care is having trouble affording health care, you should speak to the physician immediately. There may be programs or health resources in your area for patients who do not have enough money for their medical care. It's very important to be sensitive and attentive to this vulnerable portion of the community.

Major Health Problems of Specific Cultural Groups

Cultural competence takes time, practice, and skill. In addition to all you have learned about being culturally competent, there are some health issues that are specifically connected to certain cultural groups.

- Some forms of cancer are linked to certain cultural groups.
- Cardiovascular disease is seen more often in Caucasian people with average incomes.
- A blood disorder called sickle-cell anemia is seen most often in African Americans.
- Alcoholism, smoking, or suicide may be more common in certain cultural groups or in certain geographic areas.

Remember that even if certain health issues are more common in specific groups of people, it's still critically important that you approach every patient as a unique individual.

OUTCOMES

In a culturally competent office, the policies and practices that are displayed result in positive interactions for you, your coworkers, and your patients. An environment that is free of bias and stereotyping helps make patients more comfortable. An office that works hard to connect patients to the community adds further to the cultural competence of your workplace. As a result, your daily experiences as well as the experiences of every patient who comes to your office are more rewarding.

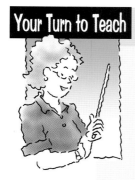

Your Turn to Teach

RISK FACTORS FOR AFRICAN AMERICANS

You know that what is true of one person may not be true of another. But it's also true that certain cultural groups are prone to certain health risks. If you're counseling an African-American patient about risk factors, here are some important facts for you to discuss.

- Young African-American men and women are at a higher risk for contracting HIV than their Caucasian or Asian peers. Medical experts are still trying to learn why this is so. But regardless of the reason, it's important for your African-American patients to know about the risks and make informed decisions about their health and safety.

- Sickle-cell anemia is an inherited blood disease. It affects the shape of red blood cells, which affects their ability to carry oxygen throughout the body. While the disease is by no means exclusive to African Americans, it does affect a larger percentage of the African-American community, or one out of every 500 African Americans.

- While Caucasian women are more likely to develop breast cancer than their African-American peers, African-American women with breast cancer are more likely to die of the disease than Caucasian women. Medical experts do not have a clear answer for why this is so. But it's important in any case for African-American women to be checked regularly for the first signs of breast cancer.

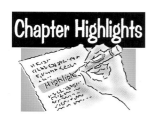

Chapter Highlights

- Your culture is the set of learned and shared beliefs, values, and expectations that you use in your social interactions with others. Cultural competence is the set of beliefs, skills, and attitudes you use to interact effectively with patients of all cultures.

- Developing policies and procedures for treating all patients with respect for their individual cultures as well as providing pamphlets and brochures in multiple languages will help create a culturally competent workplace.

- Listening, patience, acceptance, and tolerance are all skills necessary to communicate with a culturally diverse population.
- Members of some cultures may trust traditional healing practices over modern medical solutions. The members of some cultures may have strict rules for eating, fasting, or speaking with strangers of the opposite sex.
- It's essential to be aware of nonverbal communication cues and use nonverbal communication skills when communicating with patients who have limited English proficiency.
- Some health issues are the result of where people live or their economic status. For example, people living in rural communities may have limited access to health care. People living in poverty, or older adults living on fixed incomes, may have difficulty affording medical care.
- Members of specific cultural groups may be genetically predisposed to certain health conditions. However, it's critically important that you approach every patient as a unique individual.

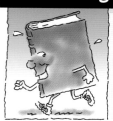

Active Learning

COMMUNICATING WITHOUT WORDS

Imagine that you're asked to escort a patient back to the examination room. The physician has also asked you to identify the reason for the patient's visit (chief complaint). However, suppose the patient does not speak any English. How would you communicate with him?

With a partner, act out the roles of non–English-speaking patient and medical assistant. Without using words, escort the patient to an "examination room" and obtain the patient's chief complaint. Then, switch roles and repeat.

Finally, share with the rest of the class the various methods you and your partner used to communicate.

CULTURAL DIFFERENCES IN DIET

Using the information presented in *Cultural Differences in Nutrition* on page 141 as a starting point, choose a culture that you know very little about and research cultural differences in diet. Create a list with two columns to identify areas in which your own culture's diet is similar to and different from the diet of the cultural group you've chosen to research.

Cultural Awareness Self-Assessment

In this chapter, you read about the importance of cultural competence. To become a culturally competent health care professional, you must have a high level of cultural awareness. How culturally aware are you? Are there areas where you need improvement? Take this short self-assessment to find out!

Directions: Enter Y for "yes" or N for "no" for each item.

___ I believe that all patients should be treated with respect for their culture, even though it may be different from my own.

___ I do not impose my beliefs and values onto patients or their family members.

___ I believe it's OK to speak a language other than English.

___ I'm aware that the roles family members play may differ according to culture.

___ I understand that male-female roles may vary among different cultures and ethnic groups, and I recognize and respect the designated decision maker in each family.

___ For patients and families who speak languages other than my own, I'll try to learn and use key words in their language so I can communicate with them better.

___ I understand that people who have limited English skills have the same intellectual capacity as anyone else and may be very capable of communicating clearly in their own language.

___ I recognize that the meaning or value of medical treatment and health education may vary greatly among cultures.

___ I understand that religion and other beliefs may affect how patients and families respond to illness, disease, and death.

___ I recognize that culture may influence verbal and nonverbal communication in many ways, including eye contact, personal space, asking and responding to questions, and comfort with silence.

____ I believe that posters, magazines, and brochures in the medical office should be of interest to and reflect the different cultures of patients and families served by a medical practice.

____ I think it's important to stay up to date on major health concerns and issues for the different ethnic groups living in the area served by a medical office.

Adapted from Goode TD. Promoting cultural competence and cultural diversity in early intervention and early childhood settings (Washington, DC: Georgetown University Center for Child and Human Development, 1989, revised 2002).

Chapter 6

TECHNIQUES TO TACKLE COMMUNICATION CHALLENGES

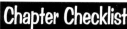

Chapter Checklist

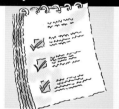

- Describe the skills a medical assistant needs to work effectively with special-needs patients

- Describe the types of patients who can be affected by drug or alcohol abuse

- Define grief

- Identify confidentiality issues related to patients with HIV/AIDS

- Describe effective ways to combat stress and anxiety

- Describe anger and its effects

- Explain how the medical assistant should act with regard to patients with disabilities

- Identify the proper procedure for reporting suspected abuse

Chapter Competencies

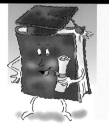

- Identify and respond to issues of confidentiality (CAAHEP Competency 3.c.2.a.)

- Maintain confidentiality at all times (ABHES Competency 1.b.)

- Use appropriate guidelines when releasing records or information (ABHES Competency 5.c.)

- Perform within legal and ethical boundaries (CAAHEP Competency 3.c.2.b.)

- Be cognizant of ethical boundaries (ABHES Competency 1.d.)
- Demonstrate knowledge of federal and state health care legislation and regulations (CAAHEP Competency 3.c.2.f.)
- Monitor legislation related to current health care issues and practices (ABHES Competency 5.g.)
- Recognize and respond to verbal and nonverbal communication (ABHES Competency 2.i., 2.k., and 2.l.; CAAHEP Competency 3.c.1.b. and 3.c.1.c.)
- Be attentive, listen, and learn (ABHES Competency 2.a.)
- Be impartial and show empathy when dealing with patients (ABHES Competency 2.b.)

In the course of your interactions with patients, you'll encounter many difficult challenges. Issues related to addiction, abuse, disabilities, depression, anger, and loss require specific communication skills. These situations present unique opportunities for you to help and support your patients in times of critical need. Being prepared for these kinds of challenges will reinforce your success as a medical assistant.

In this chapter, you'll explore in detail some special communication challenges that medical assistants face. You'll also learn the skills required to deal effectively with these challenges.

Communication Challenges

You have already learned many communication skills and techniques to use when interacting with patients of different ages and cultures. You should see by now that these skills and techniques help lay the foundation for your interactions with all patients. But, some situations with patients will present special challenges for you to face. These situations may require a specific approach and additional communication skills.

TYPES OF CHALLENGES

The following is a list of the types of special communication challenges you may face as a medical assistant. You'll explore each of these challenges separately and learn specific communication skills to use in each situation.

- patients with drug or alcohol addiction
- patients dealing with grief and loss
- HIV-positive patients
- patients with stress and anxiety
- angry and aggressive patients
- patients with disabilities
- depressed or suicidal patients
- patients who harass or abuse others

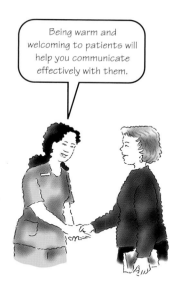

Being warm and welcoming to patients will help you communicate effectively with them.

COMMUNICATE EFFECTIVELY

By now you should understand that there are certain basic skills that make your communications with patients effective. For example, when you interact with a patient, present an open stance, listen closely, and remember that your goal is to meet the patient's health needs.

Set the Mood

Remember that your role is not to preach to, put down, or lecture patients. The patient must feel that he is being supported by you and anyone else who interacts with him. Setting the mood in the patient's environment is extremely important. Everyone and everything surrounding the patient should be comfortable, calm, soothing, and supportive.

Adapt Your Communication Style

As you have learned, the patients you see will differ in their background, age, culture, life experiences, and beliefs. You know that you should communicate with all patients with understanding and compassion. But, there are some specific ways that you'll adapt your communication style to suit a patient's unique qualities. In other words, you may say and do similar things to all patients. But *how* you say and do them will differ according to the unique qualities and situation of each patient. Learning how to adapt your communication style in this way increases your effectiveness as a medical assistant.

Drug and Alcohol Addiction

An **addiction** is a disease in which a person craves something such as alcohol or drugs and acts on those cravings, even when doing so is harmful to the person or to others. When a person is addicted, she is dependent on the object of her addiction. When a person becomes addicted to a drug or to alcohol, the addiction affects the person's ability to be and stay healthy. As you can see, interacting with a patient who has an addiction requires some very special communication skills.

UNDERSTANDING DRUG AND ALCOHOL ADDICTION

The number of people in the United States affected by drug or alcohol addiction may surprise you. In this country, 1 in 13 adults has experienced the negative effects of alcohol addiction. It's estimated that about 18 million Americans have alcohol problems, and about 5 to 6 million Americans have drug problems.

Addiction is a serious problem for addicts and nonaddicts. As a medical assistant, you may meet and work with patients who have addictions. Understanding how addictions affect a person's overall health will help you interact more effectively with her.

Health Problems of an Addict

Long-term use of drugs or alcohol has many negative effects on a person's health and behavior. For example, people who have been addicted to drugs or alcohol for a long time may have a decreased ability to behave appropriately around others. A disease called cirrhosis of the liver is commonly seen in people with a long-term addiction to alcohol. A person with a drug or alcohol addiction may also suffer from these health complications:

- malnutrition
- brain and nerve damage
- certain types of cancer
- heart disease
- liver disease
- hepatitis
- high blood pressure
- osteoporosis
- mental confusion

Anyone Can Be an Addict

You learned in an earlier chapter about the dangers of being culturally insensitive toward patients. Judging a patient because of his race, religion, culture, or any other characteristic prevents you from having effective communication. Keeping an open attitude also applies to patients with addictions. Anyone can be an addict.

It does not matter what a patient's age, profession, gender, culture, race, or religion is. It does not matter what kind of house a patient lives in, how much money a patient makes, or what the patient does for a living. Addiction has many faces, and every face is different.

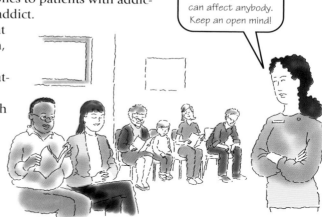

Remember, addiction can affect anybody. Keep an open mind!

Addiction Is Chronic and Progressive

Addiction is a chronic disease. It's not a temporary problem; many addicts struggle with addiction throughout their lives. Addiction is also progressive. It can become more severe over time and affect all aspects of an addict's life. A person's addiction can become the driving force behind all her social activities. For many addicts, every decision made throughout the day is driven by the need to satisfy their addiction.

There is also a financial cost of addictions—and, addicts are not the only ones who pay. Society ends up paying as well. It's estimated that every American adult pays almost $1,000 per year for damages related to addiction. In fact, untreated addiction is more expensive than heart disease, diabetes, and cancer combined.

Different Ideas About Addiction

Why does a person become addicted to alcohol or drugs? Some studies have shown that there may be a genetic link between family members who have an addiction. But, there also seem to be many cultural and environmental factors that contribute to addiction. It's probably the interaction between all of these factors that drives a person to choose to abuse alcohol or drugs.

COMMON CHARACTERISTICS OF ADDICTION

What kinds of physical characteristics might an addict have? As mentioned before, you may not necessarily be able to tell an addict from a nonaddict. But, there are some symptoms of drug and alcohol addiction that you should be on the lookout for. Here is a list of some of the symptoms:

- flushed skin
- odor on the breath
- difficulty focusing
- loss of memory
- irritability
- dilated pupils
- inflammation of whites of eyes
- depression
- behavior changes

Remember that many of these symptoms may be connected to health problems other than addiction. If you suspect a patient has an addiction to drugs or alcohol, be sure to notify the physician.

Along with the physical symptoms of addiction, addicts also have the tendency to blame others for their addiction. In fact, the first step in recognizing one's own addiction is taking responsibility for the addiction and not placing the blame on somebody else.

THERAPEUTIC TECHNIQUES

Your support and understanding has a great effect on patients who are struggling with an addiction. A patient's addiction affects everything in that patient's life, including his health. Therefore, there are some specific things to keep in mind when you respond to and communicate with a patient who is an addict.

Treat with Compassion

As always, make sure you interact with all patients with compassion and understanding. But, remember that an addict's self-esteem is usually low. Because of this, a patient with an addiction requires even more compassion and understanding.

Involve Family Members

Make sure that supportive family and friends are involved with the health of the person who is addicted. Deciding to give up alcohol or drugs is not easy for an addict. The process of withdrawal from alcohol or drugs is even more difficult and challenging. A recovering addict needs as much love and support as possible.

Suggest Support Groups

There are many organizations and help groups available to addicts. Know the names and phone numbers of community organizations, agencies, or support groups that addicts can call or contact for help. Have this information handy.

Do Not Take Relapse Personally

You may meet a patient who has a drug addiction. In the course of your interaction with the patient, you may help her with other health issues as well as help her find the resources to treat her addiction. Suppose the patient decides to stop using drugs and is successful for several months. But after five months, the patient comes into the office for a non–drug-related issue, and you suspect that she has relapsed and taken drugs recently.

It would be easy to blame yourself for the patient's relapse. But remember, all patients must take responsibility for their own health. You can offer support and information. But in the end, it's the patient who makes the decision to take or not take medication, eat healthy or unhealthy foods, exercise or not exercise, and take drugs or not take drugs.

Grief and Loss Reactions

As a medical assistant, you may be faced with providing comfort and support to patients who are terminally ill. You may also interact with patients or a patient's family members during times of grief. There are many different kinds of loss. You may think of death first, but loss of cognitive ability, physical ability, or independence are also losses for which patients or family members may grieve deeply. Your ability to communicate effectively when death or another loss occurs is important. The first step in doing this is to accept your own feelings about death and dying. It's also important to understand what the stages of grief are and what happens during each stage.

KÜBLER-ROSS—THE STAGES OF GRIEF

Elisabeth Kübler-Ross was a psychiatrist who was very interested in the treatment of terminally ill patients. In 1969, Kübler-Ross wrote a book in which she described five stages of grief that

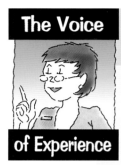

WORKING WITH PATIENTS WHO ARE ADDICTED TO DRUGS

Q: *How do I help a patient who is addicted to drugs? The patient's continuing drug use affects her health, and I do not know what to do.*

A: A patient with a drug addiction may not want to be helped. In fact, a patient who is addicted to one or more drugs may not even think she has a problem at all. A patient may come to see a physician for reasons other than those related directly to an addiction. If you strongly suspect a patient has an addiction, here are some steps you can take.

- Notify the physician immediately. The physician is in the best position to assess the patient's symptoms and offer guidance to the patient. Help the physician by collecting as much information as you can.

- Find community resources. Gather together phone numbers, names, and addresses of resources in the community that the patient or a family member can contact for help.

- Follow-up. Check back with the patient to see how he is doing and remind him of any follow-up exams with the physician.

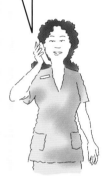

Hi, Mrs. Lee. I'm just calling to see how you're doing since we last spoke, and to remind you of your follow-up appointment.

people go through when they experience a loss. Grief is a reaction that is usually associated with the death of a loved one, but in fact can occur when we experience a loss of any kind. Terminally ill patients can experience grief when facing their own death. The five stages of grief are:

- denial
- anger
- bargaining
- depression
- acceptance

It's important to keep in mind, however, that some patients may not follow the stages in this exact order. Other patients may even go back and forth between stages before reaching the final stage, acceptance.

Denial

When a patient is in the **denial stage** of grief, the patient chooses *not* to accept that a loss will or has happened. The patient may say, "There must be a mistake" or "I do not believe it" or "I do not want to talk about it." Denial allows the patient to put distance between herself and the reality of the loss. In general, the denial stage serves three purposes.

- *Insulating from grief.* A person uses denial as protection from grief. In some cases, a loss may be so overwhelming that the person isn't ready to process what has happened. Denial delays the impact of the loss.

- *Coping with pain.* When a person experiences extreme pain, such as the pain that comes with loss, there is a tendency to isolate one's self from others. The pain associated with loss may be so great that being alone is the easiest way to cope.

- *Giving time to process.* A person in the denial stage is often overwhelmed and numb. Loss, especially sudden loss, is confusing. It takes time to sort out. The denial stage gives a person the opportunity to start to make sense of the loss.

Anger

The next stage of grief—anger—is a person's way of letting go. The patient may say, "Why me" or "This isn't fair" or "I hate this." In the **anger stage,** the patient may express extreme rage and hostility. Characteristics of this stage include:

- *Intense feelings.* A person may have intense feelings of anger or sadness and display strong behaviors.

- *Overly sensitive.* A person may react to people and situations more strongly than normal.

- *Out of control.* A person may seem to be out of control emotionally.

- *Angry at everyone.* A person may direct his anger at others, at situations, and at himself.

Bargaining

The third stage of grief is the **bargaining stage.** During this stage, a patient may try to trade or negotiate for more time. For example, a terminally ill patient might think, "If I can just make it to my daughter's wedding, I'll be satisfied. Just let me live until then." Some patients arrange wills, final wishes, family visits, or trips during this stage. Some patients may feel guilty during the bargaining stage.

Depression

During the **depression stage,** the patient goes through extreme internal grief. Depression is anger turned inward that leaves a person feeling sad and hopeless. The patient may cry for long periods and not talk much at all. Other characteristics of the depression stage include:

- *Inability to concentrate or process information.* It may be difficult or impossible for depressed patients to carry out tasks or listen carefully to conversations.
- *Lack of concern for self and surroundings.* The house may not get cleaned. Dirty dishes might sit in the sink for days. House pets may not get fed.
- *Anxiety, tension, and frustration.* A person's body language may be closed up—folded arms and/or legs, eyes looking down, shoulders slumped.

Acceptance

In the final stage of grief, the patient becomes calm and accepting. A patient has reached the **acceptance stage** when she willingly decides to deal with reality. In this stage, the patient comes to terms with loss and what it means.

KINDS OF LOSS

Loss does not always mean the death of a person. A patient may grieve the loss of an object, a job, a body part, or a situation. With any kind of loss, a person still goes through the five stages of grief.

Loss of Property

For many people, losing personal possessions is as traumatic as the loss of life. Natural disasters, crime, or accidents can result in the loss of possessions. Losing one's home, car, or personal objects may create strong feelings of grief.

Loss of Independence

As we age, we may become more dependent on others. Giving up independence can be viewed as a loss.

You're likely to witness a loss such as this when an older adult patient must be moved into a care facility. Moving from one's own home to an assisted-living home or retirement home can bring on many feel-ings of loss and grief.

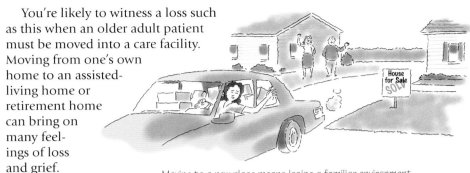

Moving to a new place means losing a familiar environment.

Loss of Body Image

When a person loses part of her body, she loses part of herself. You do not usually think of your arms, legs, hands, feet, or other body parts as being separate from *you*. They *are* you! So, if part of a patient's body must be removed for health reasons, the patient processes the loss in much the same way she would process the loss of a loved one.

You may see this kind of loss when a breast cancer patient undergoes a mastectomy. The patient will go through the grieving process as she comes to terms with the loss of part of her body.

Loss of Significant Other

The loss of a significant other is a very hard on the surviving partner. For couples who have been together for decades, the loss can seem unbearable. In some situations, family members offer support during the grieving process. But for partners who have no other family members except for the partner who is gone, the grieving process is especially difficult.

Loss of Life

Many of us first experience the grieving process because of the loss of a loved one. However, a terminally ill patient also grieves as he comes to terms with the loss of his own life. People may also grieve the loss of people they never knew. For example, people around the world grieved the loss of life after the terror-ist attacks in New York City on September 11, 2001. The loss of life associated with wars also causes many people to grieve the loss of others, even if they had never met.

UNRESOLVED GRIEF

The grieving process is different from person to person. Some people may take longer to grieve than others. Some people may get depressed, show anger, bargain, or reach acceptance in different ways than others. These differences are all normal and expected. But, serious side effects can result if a person does not go through the grieving process and her grief remains unresolved.

It's important to understand that the grieving process is normal and necessary. When it's not allowed to occur, the body and mind find other ways to resolve the grief. For example, some people may suffer from unexplained headaches, digestive problems, or other aches and pains.

Remember that you can't plan how long to grieve. There is no set time frame for the grieving process.

COMING TO TERMS WITH LOSS

As you can see, it's vitally important that people go through the grieving process after a loss. Coming to terms with a loss is part of the cycle of life and death. Along with the grieving process, here are some additional ways to help your patients come to terms with loss.

Allow Time to Grieve

Remind your patients that grieving takes time. The length of time may be different for different people. It's important not to plan on the grieving process ending at a certain time. It may not.

Talk with Others

Friends, family members, and others can be a great source of support to grieving patients. Encourage them to talk to close friends and family members. In addition, many communities have grief support groups that meet regularly. People in these groups often provide support for one another by sharing similar experiences. Have information about these groups on hand for your patients.

Postpone Major Decisions

The time your patients spend grieving is probably not the best time for them to make major decisions. For example, if at all possible, patients should put off making important life decisions such as moving, selling property, changing jobs, or making large purchases. If you suspect a patient is planning to make a major life change while he is still grieving, let the physician know.

Sleep

During sleep, the body and mind heal, rest, and renew. Although patients might find it difficult to sleep while going through a grieving process, it's still important that they try to sleep as normally as possible. Tell your patients that taking naps or lying down for brief periods throughout the day may help.

Lower Self-Expectations

The grieving process requires energy just as any other body process does. In fact, it requires more energy than people are aware of. Therefore, trying to function normally (in work, at home, with friends, and with hobbies) while grieving is unrealistic. Let your patients know that they can't do it all. And that's okay.

THERAPEUTIC COMMUNICATION TECHNIQUES

There are many ways that you, as a medical assistant, can communicate effectively with a patient who is grieving. Use the skills you have already practiced and learned, and remember that each person is an individual. Here is a list of communication techniques to keep in mind:

- *Listen.* Pay attention to what the patient is saying.
- *Empathy.* Treat each patient with compassion and understanding.
- *Structure.* Identify the patient's specific concerns.
- *Support.* Allow the patient time to grieve.

Each Patient Is an Individual

You know that every patient is an individual. Two patients with the same illness would probably describe how they are feeling in two different ways. In the same way, every person grieves in his own way. There is no "correct" way to grieve. It's important that you remember to treat each patient as an individual, respecting the way he chooses to grieve.

Listen

As always, be sure to listen to what your patients have to say. During the grieving process, it's often difficult for people to express how they are feeling. Be patient. Allow the patient time to speak. Use all you have learned about communication to help the patient express what she needs to express.

Let Patients Express Themselves

Some patients may need nothing more than someone to listen to them talk. Expressing how they feel and think about death or life may be a critical need for some patients. If so, your job is to listen sincerely and attentively. You may have past experiences with grieving, but this may not be the time to share them. Try to focus on what the patient needs to express, and do not be afraid of long periods of silence.

Recognize Nonverbal Messages

Watch the patient's body language and facial expressions for nonverbal messages. During the grieving process, a patient may say more with her body and face than at other times.

In some cases, you may find that a patient prefers not to speak at all. In this case, offer a warm hand gesture or a soothing smile to let the patient know you understand and care.

Ask How You Can Help

If you do not know what to do or say, simply ask, "What can I do to help you?" A patient who is grieving may need nothing more than a hug, a smile, a gentle squeeze of the shoulder, or maybe just a few moments alone. The important thing is to ask.

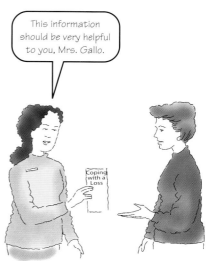

What can I do to help you?

Provide Empathy and Support

Let the patient know that you care about his feelings. Some patients want to be reassured that they are not alone in their grief. If you sense a patient needs to talk about how others have coped with grief, go ahead and share a personal experience, or offer the patient information about community groups for coping with grief. Let the patient know that you empathize.

Make Patients Feel Comfortable

Use what you have learned to make patients feel comfortable. By doing this, you'll be giving patients a safe environment in which to express their feelings and emotions freely.

This information should be very helpful to you, Mrs. Gallo.

Be Honest

Explain in simple yet basic terms what you know about death and dying. Give patients pamphlets of other information you have on the subject. Let patients know what they can expect. Present information in a professional but basic manner. Patients appreciate being told things honestly, even when the information is difficult to hear.

Coping with a Loss

Be Open

Allow patients to share what they are feeling and thinking. Use your body language to let patients know that you're approachable and happy to listen. When you do this, you send the message that you're there to help the patient feel better.

Identify Concerns

Identify the specific concerns of the patient. Some patients may be upset or concerned about issues outside the grieving process. Find out what these specific concerns are. Ask the patient to share specific concerns with you.

Allow Time to Grieve

As mentioned earlier, be sure to give patients time to grieve, to speak, to think, and to feel. Resolving the issue of loss does not happen easily or quickly.

HIV/AIDS

Since 1981, the disease known as **AIDS** has become one of the most serious health threats in history. AIDS is a deadly disease that is caused by a virus called **HIV.** There is no cure for AIDS.

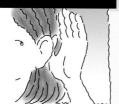

Listen to This

STAGES OF GRIEF AND LOSS

Here are some suggestions for communicating with patients who are in or about to be in any of the stages of grief.

- Let the person talk. Listen without interrupting.
- Let the person show all their feelings. A person who is grieving may cry, laugh, or shout in one conversation.
- Give the person as much time as he needs.
- Ask what you can do to help.
- If the person does not know how you can help, offer suggestions.
- If the person would welcome a hug or handclasp, do it. However, be culturally sensitive—touching may not be appropriate.
- Suggest a support group.
- Provide resources for counseling if the physician recommends counseling.

As the incidence of AIDS continues to go up, the probability increases that you'll meet and work with patients who are either infected with HIV (HIV positive) or who have AIDS. Therefore, it's important that you learn as much information as possible about AIDS and HIV to increase your awareness.

AIDS

AIDS stands for acquired immunodeficiency syndrome. *Acquired* means that the disease is contracted from something or someone else. *Immunodeficiency* means that the disease targets a person's immune system and makes it weaker. *Syndrome* means that the disease has many symptoms that occur together. When a person has AIDS, her immune system becomes so weakened that it can no longer do its job to protect the body against infection. As a result, the person suffers from many infections that a healthy body could easily fight off. In a person with AIDS, simple infections can become life threatening.

International Health Care Crisis

The spread of HIV and AIDS has become so serious that it's considered an international health care crisis. The rate of HIV infection is still increasing around the world. In developing nations, the rate of death from AIDS is doubling and, in some cases, tripling. HIV can be transmitted in any country and on any continent.

Educating people about HIV and AIDS and improving health care will help control the crisis. Scientists and doctors are constantly developing new ways to treat and prevent the disease.

What Causes AIDS?

AIDS is caused by a retrovirus called HIV. HIV stands for human immunodeficiency virus. When a person is infected with HIV, the virus invades special white blood cells, called helper T cells, in the immune system. The immune system helps a person's body fight off infection and prevent disease. When HIV invades helper T cells, the person's immune system begins to weaken. A blood test can determine whether a person is HIV positive, meaning that the person has been infected with HIV, or HIV negative.

THERAPEUTIC COMMUNICATION TECHNIQUES

There are many issues to keep in mind when communicating with a patient who is HIV positive or has AIDS. Misunderstanding and misinformation about HIV and AIDS are still a big problem. Because of this, your knowledge, understanding, support, and communication skills are vitally important.

Know the Facts About HIV/AIDS

It's your responsibility as a medical assistant to be educated about HIV and AIDS. Knowing how the virus is spread, the way that HIV invades the immune system, the symptoms of AIDS, and how AIDS progresses will help you approach HIV and AIDS with intelligence, compassion, and understanding. It will also better prepare you to work with all patients, including those who are HIV positive or have AIDS.

Examine Your Feelings About HIV/AIDS

It's important to examine your own feelings about HIV and AIDS. How do you feel about the HIV/AIDS crisis? What will your feelings be toward patients who might be HIV positive? How would you feel about working with patients with AIDS? Examine your answers to these and other questions. Talk with others if necessary. As in other situations, make sure you're prepared to give equal care and attention to all patients.

Examine Your Feelings About Dying

Unfortunately, many people with HIV/AIDS die at a relatively young age. Because of this, make sure that you have closely examined your own feelings about death and dying. Research the topics of AIDS, death, grieving, and loss. Seek out other resources that can help you resolve any issues you have about death and dying.

Establish a Supportive Environment

A patient with HIV or AIDS must deal with many issues and emotions. When working with these patients, as with all patients, be prepared to listen and to offer support. A person who has AIDS may lose their job. They may feel guilty for having AIDS. They may feel shame and embarrassment. They may have lost friends and the support of family members. As much as you're able, give the HIV/AIDS patient all the support and empathy you can.

LEGAL CONSIDERATIONS

Since many people still do not understand how HIV is spread or what AIDS is, much misunderstanding exists. To protect the dignity and personal rights of people with AIDS, there are certain legal considerations to keep in mind. As a medical assistant, make sure you're aware of the following considerations:

Informed Consent for HIV Testing

There are several legal issues to consider when testing for HIV. The laws in each state vary. But, one issue on which all states agree is that a patient must sign an informed consent form before being tested for HIV. Make sure you're familiar with these forms and can easily explain what they are to patients.

Laws of Confidentiality

To keep the details of any HIV test confidential, most laboratories will use a number or other coding system, rather than the patient's name, to identify blood samples.

As a medical assistant, you need to know whether a patient is HIV positive or not. The physician, of course, will also need to know this information. Other patients definitely should not be made aware of this or any other information in the patient's medical record. Make sure all patients, including patients with HIV or AIDS, feel safe and respected. The patient's rights to privacy and confidentiality are important.

State Reporting Guidelines

Laboratories that do HIV testing must be approved by the state for such testing. Also, most laws are very specific about when, how, and to whom HIV test results can be given. Make sure you comply with the reporting guidelines in your state.

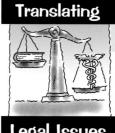
Translating
Legal Issues

LEGAL RIGHTS FOR PATIENTS WITH HIV OR AIDS

In most states, a person who has HIV or AIDS is guaranteed equal rights to employment, education, privacy, shelter, and health care. The following is a summary of those rights:

- A person can't refuse to rent an apartment or home to a person who has HIV/AIDS.
- A restaurant or hotel can't refuse service to a person who has HIV/AIDS.
- A public place can't refuse service to a person who has HIV/AIDS.
- An employer can't refuse to hire a person because he or she has HIV/AIDS.
- An employer can't require a person to take an HIV test before deciding to hire that person.

Stress and Anxiety

Stress is a condition that happens when a change in a person's environment is felt as a challenge, a threat, or a danger. Stress can produce negative or positive results. Stress is a part of everyone's lives. But, the way you react to stress may be different from the way another person responds to the same stress.

You'll work with patients who are experiencing various levels of stress and anxiety. It's important that you understand these feelings and learn how to communicate effectively and interact with patients who are stressed and anxious.

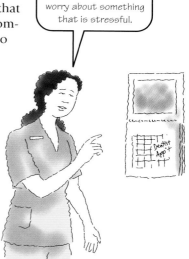

Anxiety is a feeling of worry about something that is stressful.

ANXIETY

Many people have anxiety when they experience stress. **Anxiety** is an emotional state in which people feel uneasy, apprehensive, or fearful. Someone with anxiety may feel worried or nervous about something that is going to happen.

In many cases, anxiety and stress go together. Suppose you have a dentist appointment and you do not like going to the dentist. In this case, having to go to the dentist is stressful. The feeling of dread you have about going to the dentist is the anxiety you feel about the stress.

SYMPTOMS OF STRESS AND ANXIETY

You may not always know when you're experiencing stress and anxiety. Sometimes, it takes an outsider to observe what you're doing and saying. In the same way, knowing the symptoms of stress and anxiety can help you identify a patient who is stressed and anxious. The symptoms of stress and anxiety can be divided into low-level or high-level symptoms.

Low-Level Symptoms

People usually feel anxious about something they can't control, change, or predict. Something that seems threatening or dangerous can also bring about feelings of anxiety. Some low-level symptoms you might observe in a patient who is stressed or anxious include:

- fidgeting
- muscle tension

- sleeping problems
- headache

High-Level Symptoms

When the stress is more serious, or when the patient is having difficulty coping with a stressful situation, you may observe high-level symptoms. High-level symptoms of stress and anxiety include:

- rapid heartbeat
- sweating
- increased blood pressure
- nausea
- dizziness

THERAPEUTIC TECHNIQUES

Interacting with patients who are stressed is a challenge that you'll encounter often. For yourself and for your patients, always remember this: the best way to cope with stress is to live a healthy lifestyle. It's much easier for a healthy body than it is for an unhealthy body to handle stress.

When you meet a patient who is stressed or anxious, there are several stress management techniques you can suggest.

Stress Management Techniques

Remind patients that learning how to manage stress effectively involves skills that must be practiced regularly. A lifestyle that includes regular exercise, proper nutrition, and sufficient rest will help a person more effectively deal with stress.

Exercise

There is no better or healthier way to lessen the effects of stress than to exercise. Regular exercise increases circulation and keeps the mind and body toned and fit. Even for patients who do not exercise regularly, a brisk walk or other light exercise can have an immediate, positive effect.

Proper Nutrition

A balanced diet helps people feel better and makes it easier for their bodies to stay healthy. When people are stressed, their diet is usually one of the first things to suffer. Emphasize to patients that eating healthfully while they are stressed is just as important as eating healthfully when they are not stressed.

Proper Rest

As mentioned before, getting enough rest gives the body a chance to relax and renew itself. The body uses more energy when a person is stressed. Remind patients that getting enough sleep is always important, especially during stressful times.

Express Fears and Worries

Another technique that helps patients cope with stress is to let them talk about their fears and worries. Present a nonjudgmental environment so that patients feel comfortable expressing their thoughts and concerns. Patients often feel better after they have put their feelings into words. And, sharing these feelings with others usually has an instant, positive result.

Relaxation Techniques

Learning how to relax is a valuable tool for coping with stress. Help patients with different relaxation techniques. Here are three basic ways to relax:

- *Breathing.* Instruct the patient to take several slow deep breaths. Emphasize controlling the breath and breathing deeply from the abdomen.
- *Visualization.* Instruct the patient to find a quiet, soothing location and to focus on positive, relaxing situations. This is a little like daydreaming.
- *Physical exercise.* Encourage the patient to find some physical activity that she will enjoy doing regularly. Possibilities include swimming, walking, bicycling, or gardening.

Anger and Aggression

Anger is a strong feeling of displeasure or unhappiness. Sometimes, anger leads to physical violence. As a medical assistant, you should always be prepared to deal effectively with a patient who becomes angry. The best way to do this is to understand why and how anger occurs and to know how to deal with it.

ANGER IS A NATURAL EMOTION

There are many reasons for feeling angry. You might feel angry when you hear sad or upsetting news. You might get angry when somebody says or does something upsetting. The important thing to remember is that anger is a natural human emotion.

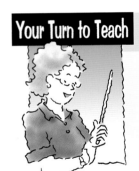

Your Turn to Teach   DEEP BREATHING

We breathe so that we can take oxygen into our bodies and release carbon dioxide, a waste product. Every time you inhale, oxygen is taken into your body, absorbed by your blood, and carried to your body cells. The deeper the breath, the more oxygen you inhale, and the more waste product you exhale. Here is a simple deep breathing technique that will increase the effectiveness of the breath.

1. Sit up straight with hands placed on the abdomen.
2. Take a deep, slow breath in through the nose.
3. Imagine the air filling your abdomen first, and then your chest, like a balloon.
4. Feel your hands being pushed away from your abdomen.
5. Hold the breath for a few seconds.
6. Exhale through the mouth with a "whooooo" sound.
7. Feel your hands being pulled in toward the abdomen.

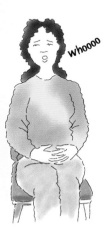

Everyone Can Feel Angry

Everyone feels angry at certain times. It's important to understand that anger, as an emotion, is not wrong. It's what people do with their anger that can become problematic.

Anger Is Often Temporary

Anger can come and go suddenly. You might be chatting nicely and calmly with a patient one minute. Then, the next minute, the patient might raise her voice at you. Emotions can change quickly when people become frustrated, disappointed, or surprised. It's not uncommon for a patient, upon hearing upsetting news about her health, to experience sadness, anger, and depression all within a very short period of time.

What Causes Anger?

A person might become angry when she feels threatened or fearful about something or someone. Some unexpected news, a surprising comment, a threatening gesture—these are the kinds of things that can make a person feel angry. Sometimes, a person might get angry as an immediate reaction to something or someone. Other times, she might stew for a long time about something and work herself into an angry state.

Where Is Anger Directed?

Anger is often directed toward a specific person or situation. If a person feels that another person or a situation is the cause of her unhappiness, it's easy to get angry and place blame. The person can even get angry at herself. If a person has just found out that she has a serious illness, she might get very angry at herself for not living more healthfully.

Managing Anger

As mentioned already, it's what people do with their anger that is really important. Anger is a normal human emotion. But, becoming physically violent and threatening others are not appropriate reactions. Anger is only a problem when people express it inappropriately.

Recognizing anger and doing something about it are critical. If anger is not managed the right way, it can lead to aggression and even violence. Violent behavior is never okay.

RECOGNIZING ANGER

How do you know when a person is angry? Fortunately, there are some very clear signs that can indicate anger in you or somebody else. These signs include:

- loud and sharp tone of voice
- tense facial expressions
- punctuated gestures
- sarcasm and criticism
- threats

Tone of Voice

When people get angry, they are upset and they may want to be heard. As a result, their tone of voice may become sharp and loud. For example, let's suppose a patient is waiting in the waiting room for an appointment. After waiting for quite a long time, she finally raises her voice in anger and says, "Am I going to wait much longer?" Because of the woman's tone, she immediately gets the attention of the receptionist, who says, "It will be just a few minutes longer."

Facial Expressions

Not all people use words to show their anger. In some cases, the only way you know that a person is angry is by looking at her facial expression. It's common for an angry person to be red-faced. An angry person may avoid making eye contact. Her eyes may be sharp, and her forehead may be tense. Her mouth may be tense and tight.

Gestures

Anger uses a lot of energy. When some people are angry, they use a lot of physical gestures to help express their anger. Arm-waving, finger-pointing, and fist-clenching are common gestures seen with anger.

Sarcasm and Criticism

When people are angry, they may lash out at others using sarcasm and criticism. Putting down, criticizing, and insulting others are all ways of expressing angry feelings. Unfortunately, these kinds of comments are hurtful and make it hard for others to want to help the angry person.

Threats

Sometimes, if anger is not responded to in the desired manner, a person will resort to threats. Let's look again at the example of the angry patient waiting for her appointment. If nobody responds to the patient's voice or gestures, she might then resort to making a threat such as, "If somebody does not get me in to see a physician now, I'm going to go find the physician myself!"

THERAPEUTIC COMMUNICATION TECHNIQUES

As you have probably guessed by now, learning how to manage patients who are angry can be a valuable skill. There are several things you can do as a medical assistant to prevent, decrease, or calm anger before it gets out of hand.

Let Patients Express Themselves

Getting to the real cause of the anger is often a key step in calming an angry person. First, help the patient admit that she is angry. Then, help the patient put into words the exact reason for her anger. Encourage the patient to put her feelings into her own words.

Do Not Take Things Personally

People say things in anger that are often cruel and hurtful. Do not take these comments personally. A person who is angry may say things to get attention. He may make exaggerated state-

ments, say things that are very mean, or blurt out wild comments just to be recognized.

Attempt to Understand

Let the patient know that you want to understand why she is
angry. Keep your voice as calm as possible. Keep your body language controlled. Contrast the patient's anger by being cool and
calm. Make eye contact and say to the patient, "Help me understand why you're feeling angry."

Recognize Verbal and Nonverbal Cues

Being able to spot anger quickly is an especially helpful
skill. Observing certain facial expressions and body language may indicate that a patient is becoming frustrated. Approaching and interacting with the patient
before she becomes angry can prevent the situation
from getting out of hand. Therefore, recognizing
verbal and nonverbal cues of anger is very important.

Let's go into this other room where you can tell me what the problem is.

Attempt to De-Escalate

One of the quickest ways to calm down, or de-
escalate, an angry patient is to change her environment. If a patient is displaying disruptive
angry behavior in the waiting room of your office,
quickly bring that patient into another room where
you can speak to her privately.

Let Patients Communicate Emotions

Allow the patient time to express her feelings and emotions to you. As you know by now, listening is one of the most
important communication skills you can use with patients. It's
even more important with patients who are angry. A patient
who is angry usually wants to be heard NOW!

Find the Source of Anger

The first step in being able to manage anger effectively is to know
why a person is angry in the first place. Being able to identify the
source of anger makes it easier to prevent anger from happening
in the future. If, for example, waiting more than 15 minutes for an
appointment makes a patient angry, the receptionist can make the
patient's next appointment for a day and time that is not so busy.

Identify Triggers

Certain topics and situations may make certain people angry.
Try to find out what these triggers are. Think of ways to change
the trigger or get rid of it altogether. Maybe you tend to get angry

more quickly if you're hungry. If this is the case, make sure you have a meal or grab a light snack before coming to work.

Think About Consequences

What happens when people get angry? In most situations, anger is disruptive, and people's feelings can get hurt. Most people end up apologizing for their angry outburst or display. Relationships may be harmed or even destroyed by anger. It's difficult to think rationally about consequences in the midst of anger. So, it makes more sense to think about the consequences beforehand. If you tend to get angry at family members, coworkers, or others, think about what happens when you show signs of anger. How often does getting angry get you what you really need? When working with patients, often getting angry is the least effective way to get to the solution or conclusion you need.

Relaxation and Exercise

Two of the best ways to manage anger are by practicing relaxation techniques and exercising. Tell your patients about these useful techniques. Also, use these techniques to help keep yourself calm. Get into the habit of practicing relaxation and deep breathing. When you're used to relaxing on a regular basis, it will be easier to do so to calm your anger.

Exercise or other physical activity is a quick way to stop anger in its tracks. If you start to feel angry, leave the room and take a quick walk around the building. Go to the gym for a workout. Do a quick set of sit-ups or push-ups. Physical activity is a great way to use energy effectively.

Disabilities

Another communication challenge is working with patients who have disabilities. A **disability** is something that restricts a person's major life activities. When working with patients with disabilities, you must be able to determine how the patient's disability affects his ability to communicate. In some cases, a friend, caregiver, or family member will be present to help. Make sure that, whatever the disability, you include the patient in the communication process. As with all patients, help make patients with disabilities feel that they are taking part in their own health care.

TYPES OF IMPAIRMENTS

A person with a disability may have one or more impairments. An **impairment** is something that weakens or lessens the effectiveness of something else. A person may be physically disabled because of

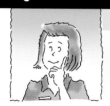

Say it Isn't So

WHAT HAPPENS WHEN A PATIENT IS ANGRY?

What if a patient becomes angry? What are some helpful ways of interacting with the patient?

Suppose you meet a patient, Mr. Patel, who complains about everything and everyone in the office. He makes very little eye contact with anybody and is visibly angry. You can see that Mr. Patel is furious about something. What should you do?

Anger is often a mask for fear. Knowing this will guide you in your interactions with any angry patient. The most important strategy when working with a patient who is angry is to keep your interaction centered on the patient and his feelings. Ask Mr. Patel, "How are you feeling?" Find out why Mr. Patel is feeling angry by asking, "Can you tell me what is making you feel angry?" Do not be afraid to get to the bottom of the patient's feelings. It's equally important to know that if a patient becomes disrespectful or threatening, you should immediately leave the room and ask your supervisor or the physician for assistance.

a visual impairment, hearing impairment, speaking impairment, or some other physical impairment. Or a person may be developmentally disabled because of a mental impairment.

Mobility Impairments

When an impairment affects a person's mobility, it makes it harder for the person to get from place to place. Patients with a physical impairment may have one or more artificial limb or may be paralyzed. Some may use a wheelchair. Remember that a patient's wheelchair is part of that patient. Treat it and the patient with respect and dignity.

Visual Impairments and Blindness

Patients who are disabled because of visual impairments may have limited or no vision. A patient who has trouble seeing will not pick up on nonverbal messages and cues. Some patients with a visual impairment wear special glasses or use a special walking cane. For some patients, such as those with macular degeneration, only certain areas in their field of vision are impaired. Center yourself in front of the patient, and do not move around unless it's necessary.

Hearing Impairments

Patients with a hearing impairment may not hear well or at all. Some may wear a hearing aid. Hearing loss may mean that the person can't hear high-frequency sounds. Some may rely on lip-reading. Others may use ASL (American Sign Language) or other visually based languages. If you're not familiar with the visually based language a patient is using, you can rely on written notes for communication. Keep these things in mind when communicating with these patients.

Developmental Disabilities

A developmental disability is one that affects a person before he becomes an adult. It's something that prevents the person from reaching certain developmental milestones. The person's mental and/or physical function may be affected. It's common for a person who is developmentally disabled to have some physical impairments as well. It's important to know and remember that people with developmental disabilities have the same physical and emotional needs as everyone else.

THERAPEUTIC COMMUNICATION TECHNIQUES

Some communication techniques are used only with people with certain impairments. Some techniques are used with all patients with disabilities. A technique that applies to all cases is to speak clearly, distinctly, and directly to the patient.

For each of the sections below, there is a bulleted list of communication tips to use when working with patients who have a specific disability.

Patients Who Have Artificial Limbs

- Offer to shake hands. People with limited hand use or an artificial limb can usually shake hands. Shaking with the left hand is okay.
- People with artificial legs may need extra time to move from place to place. Be careful not to rush them.
- Ask the patient if he needs extra help. Many people with artificial limbs prefer doing things on their own first. So, ask before helping.

Patients Who Are Visually Impaired

- Use a normal tone of voice. There is no reason to raise your voice.

- Let the patient know you're in the room.
- Explain any sounds or movements that might confuse or concern the patient.
- Identify yourself and anybody else who might be with you.
- Offer assistance and help the patient only after the offer is accepted. Do not say, "Here let me help you onto the examination table" *while* you're helping the patient onto the table. Wait for the patient to accept your offer. Then ask the patient to explain how you can help.

Patients in Wheelchairs

- Remember that the wheelchair is part of the patient's personal space.
- Never lean on a patient's wheelchair.
- Do not assume a patient wants you to push his wheelchair. Ask first.

Patients Who Are Speech Impaired

- Listen attentively.
- Give feedback to help clarify what has been said.
- Give the patient time to speak. Be patient!

Patients Who Are Hearing Impaired

- As with the visually impaired patient, let the patient who is hearing impaired know when you're in the room.
- Tap the patient's shoulder or wave your hand to get their attention.
- Make sure the patient sees you before you start talking.
- Use a visually based language if you and the patient both know it.
- Use many nonverbal cues.
- Write down lengthy messages or instructions.
- Many people with hearing impairments can't hear high pitches. Also, hearing aids can distort high-pitched sounds. So try using a lower voice.

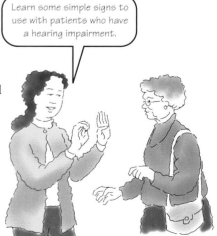

Learn some simple signs to use with patients who have a hearing impairment.

Patients with Developmental Disabilities

- Treat all patients respectfully and at a level appropriate to their developmental level of understanding.
- Maintain eye contact and always speak directly to the patient.
- Make sure there are no distractions.
- Be patient with the patient!

Depression and Suicidal Feelings

Patients who are depressed and/or suicidal may present a challenge to the medical assistant. Understanding the causes and symptoms of depression is the first step in learning how to work with patients who are depressed or suicidal. Being able to interact with these patients may be one of your toughest challenges.

DEPRESSION

Depression is a feeling of extreme sadness or hopelessness. There are many possible causes of depression. Events like the loss of a loved one, a sudden traumatic event, the loss of a job, or the loss of possessions can cause depression. However, depression is not always brought on by an event. An imbalance of certain chemicals in the brain can also cause depression.

Characteristics of Depression

In some cases, a person may need to talk to a counselor or take medication to help them through a depressive period. In many people, the painful feelings of depression go away over time. Depression that does not go away is called *clinical* depression. Clinical depression is one of the most common mental illnesses, and it affects over 19 million people in the United States every year. Women become clinically depressed about twice as often as men. Clinical depression is also common among older adults.

The most common characteristic seen in people with depression is an overall feeling of hopelessness. Depression can also make a person feel helpless, worthless, angry, and frustrated. Depression can make a person lose interest in activities that normally bring pleasure and enjoyment.

Signs of Depression

Before you can help a patient who is depressed, you must be able to recognize depression. There are several signs that might indicate that a person is depressed. A description of each one is on pages 196–197.

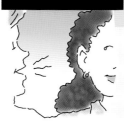

Send and Receive

THERAPEUTIC RESPONSES TO INDIVIDUALS WITH DISABILITIES

Suppose you're about to meet a patient, Mr. Levy. Mr. Levy is visually impaired and can't see. What are some communication techniques you would use with Mr. Levy? What are some things you would definitely avoid when talking with Mr. Levy? Here is an example of ineffective and effective dialogue that might take place.

Ineffective:

- After exchanging some everyday chitchat, you ask the patient, "So, what seems to be the problem today, Mr. Levy?"
- The patient answers, "Well, I'm having some pain in my knee. It's kind of hard to move it sometimes."
- You reply, "Okay. First, go ahead and get up onto the examination table." You point to the table. The patient feels around for the table before sitting on it.
- "Now, Mr. Levy, is it this knee?" You point to the patient's right knee. "Or that knee?" You point to the patient's left knee.
- Mr. Levy replies, "It's my left knee."
- "And what kind of movement makes the knee hurt?" You demonstrate using your own leg. "Does this kind of movement make it hurt? Or this kind of movement?"

In most situations you use both verbal and nonverbal methods of communicating. But with patients with visual impairments, you must remember that nonverbal cues and messages will be lost. Use only verbal cues. Let the patient touch or feel things to help get the message across.

Effective:

- After exchanging some everyday chitchat, you ask the patient, "So what seems to be the problem today, Mr. Levy?"
- The patient answers, "Well, I'm having some pain in my knee. It's kind of hard to move it sometimes."
- You reply, "Okay. First, go ahead and get up onto the examination table." You place the patient's hand on the table so he knows where it is. Mr. Levy sits on the table.

- "Now, Mr. Levy, which knee is it? And can you show me where the knee hurts?"

- Mr. Levy points to the front of his left knee. "It's here."

- "And can you describe for me the kinds of movements that make the knee hurt?"

When a patient has limited or no vision, beginning sentences with "Show me," "Tell me about, "or "Describe for me," allow you to work around the nonverbal parts of the message. Also, remember to explain your movements and any sounds for the patient.

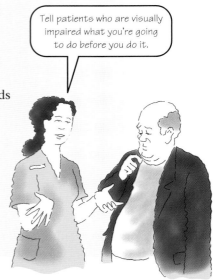

Tell patients who are visually impaired what you're going to do before you do it.

Change in Appetite

A change in eating habits is common in people who are depressed. Some people eat more when they are depressed. Some people eat less or not at all. In many cases, depression makes the physical act of eating seem like a chore. If you suspect that a patient is depressed, you might ask, "Have your eating habits changed recently?" Also, note any recent changes in weight.

Sleep Problems

Depression may cause sleeping patterns to change. People who are depressed may sleep too much or too little. When they are able to sleep at all, they may sleep restlessly. Ask a patient who you think is suffering from depression, "How are you sleeping?" Also, observe the patient's energy level. Does the patient appear tired and worn out?

Loss of Energy

One of the most common signs of depression is a loss of energy. People who are depressed complain that they have no energy to do anything. Because of this loss of energy, everyday tasks do not get done. Personal hygiene may suffer. Household chores may also be neglected. If you think a patient is suffering from clinical depression, ask, "What activities have you done this week?" This will give you an idea about the patient's energy level.

Poor Concentration

Depression can make it very difficult to concentrate for any length of time. Often, people who are depressed miss work or perform poorly at work because they can't stay focused on any one task. You may notice this lack of concentration when you speak with a patient who is depressed. The patient's body language and poor eye contact may be clues that the patient is not able to concentrate on what you're saying.

Mood Swings

People who are depressed may frequently and suddenly change moods. The person may be nervous and irritable one minute, and crying the next. They may become angry at something you say, and then start crying about their anger. In many cases, the person is overwhelmed by feelings of guilt. If you think a patient is depressed, ask, "How do you feel right now?"

Crying

It's not uncommon for people who are depressed to cry. When a person is filled with hopelessness, guilt, and sadness, crying is a logical response. Patients who are depressed may start crying as you talk to them. Or they may cry in the waiting room.

Therapeutic Communication Techniques

There are some specific ways you can help patients who are depressed. Remember, as a medical assistant, your goal is to meet the health care needs of patients. Depression is a mental illness. This means that patients suffering from depression need your support and understanding just as any other patient does.

Create a Nonthreatening Environment

The first step in meeting the needs of a patient who is depressed is to provide an environment in which the patient feels secure and comfortable. Find a quiet, private place for the patient. Make sure there are plenty of tissues. Have someone stay with the patient or check in on the patient frequently.

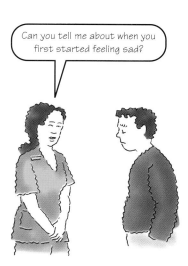

Help the Patient Identify Feelings

If possible, help the patient identify what she is feeling. Try to get the patient to name each feeling she has. Help the patient identify situations that may trigger her depression. Ask the patient if she knows what is causing each of her feelings. Sometimes, having the patient go through this process of identification will help her feel more in control of the situation.

Present Activity Options

There are several activities that can help the patient deal with depression, such as yoga, music therapy, relaxation exercises, deep breathing, and writing. Community centers usually have information about these kinds of activities. Have a list of phone numbers and names handy.

SUICIDE

A person who is depressed or has another mental illness may be considering suicide. In fact, depression is a contributing factor in most suicides or suicide attempts. As a medical assistant, you can help prevent suicide by learning how to identify depression and suicidal tendencies in your patients. To do this, you must be familiar with the warning signs of suicide, including:

- talking about suicide
- giving away possessions or making a will
- buying a weapon
- mixing drugs and alcohol

Keep in mind that any one of these signs does not necessarily indicate that a person is suicidal. Consider all factors and signs as a whole.

If you suspect a patient to be suicidal, your first step should be to notify the physician in charge immediately. When communicating with the patient, remember the following:

- Take any suicide attempt or talk about a suicide attempt seriously. The patient may joke about it, cry about it, hint at it, or simply mention it in casual conversation.
- Focus on prevention. Ask the patient, "What can I do to help?"
- Always listen and always encourage the patient to share his feelings.
- Express empathy and let the patient know he is not alone.
- Look for suicide risk factors. Consider the patient's situation, living conditions, profession, dependents, friends,

and any other details about his life that might contribute to his state of mind.

- Keep your voice calm and caring. Maintain constant eye contact. Let the patient know you care and want to help.

Witnessing the results of abuse can be emotionally difficult for medical professionals. Talk with your supervisor or the physician for advice on how to handle it.

Abuse and Harassment

As a medical assistant, you should be prepared to deal with the following challenging situations: a patient who harasses or who is abusive, as well as a patient who is the victim of abuse or harassment.

Abuse is the purposeful act of hurting another person. Abuse can be the result of something that is done to another person, or something vital that is withheld, such as food. **Harassment** is any annoying or stressful comment or behavior that is known to be unwelcome. In some cases, harassment may turn into abuse.

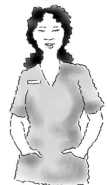

FORMS OF ABUSE

Abuse can be physical, psychological, or sexual in nature. Often more than one form of abuse is happening at the same time. Physical, psychological, and sexual abuse affect a person's body and mind. But, a person's property and personal possessions can also be abused. Abuse can also take the form of neglect. All abuse is hurtful. The victims of abuse may suffer physically, emotionally, or both.

Physical

Physical abuse causes injury to the victim's body. Slapping, biting, shaking, rough handling, and hitting are examples of physical abuse. Children and older adults are often targets of physical abuse. The physical abuse of infants is especially dangerous as it can easily result in the death of the victim. Any person whose body or state of health is weak is especially vulnerable to the effects of physical abuse.

Psychological or Emotional

There are many ways for a person to be abused psychologically or emotionally. Making a person fearful by saying cruel things or by threatening the person are examples. Hurtful statements such as "I hate you" or "You're so stupid" or "I wish you had never been born" are abusive statements.

Isolating a person from the outside world is another form of psychological abuse. A person who is rarely or never allowed to go outside and see friends or family members is being abused. Even more serious are cases in which a child or person is kept in a locked closet or other small room for long periods of time. As you can imagine, the damage from such traumatic events can last a lifetime.

Neglect

Failing to provide necessities for another person in your care is a form of abuse known as **neglect.** For example, failing to reposition a person who is bedridden is an example of neglect. People who are confined to a bed can develop sores on their body if their position is not changed regularly.

Not providing enough food or drink to another person is also neglect. Children suffer from neglect when their parent, guardian, or caregiver does not feed, clothe, or provide a safe and sanitary environment for them.

Remember that neglect is just as serious as any other form of abuse. If you suspect a patient is a victim of neglect, handle the situation just as you would any case of abuse.

Sexual

Hurtful acts that are sexual in nature are considered sexual abuse. Unwelcome comments and behaviors that are sexual in nature are considered sexual harassment. Both sexual abuse and sexual harassment can be very damaging to the victim.

Sexual Abuse

Sexual abuse happens when a person is forced to participate in sexual activity. Sexual abuse includes incest, molestation, exhibitionism, child pornography, child prostitution, and pedophilia. Some indications of sexual abuse in children include:

- withdrawn or aggressive behavior
- unusual fear of certain people or places
- sexual play or sexual drawings
- complaints of pain when going to the bathroom
- injury to the genitals
- symptoms of a sexually transmitted disease

If you suspect that a patient is a victim of sexual abuse, notify the physician immediately. Your office should have policies in place for dealing with such cases.

Sexual Harassment

Sexual harassment is any unwelcome sexual advance or request for sexual favors. In some cases, sexual harassment leads to sexual abuse. Examples of behaviors considered to be sexual harassment include:

- sexual jokes
- unwelcome gender-based behavior
- sexual bantering
- offensive pictures and language
- sexual suggestions
- suggestive behavior

You may suspect a patient of being a victim of sexual harassment. Or, you or someone you work with may be a victim of sexual harassment. In either case, your office should have policies in place for handling such situations.

Material

Material abuse includes situations in which a person's personal property or possessions are mistreated or stolen. The value of the property or possession is not important. It's never acceptable for a person to take or destroy something that belongs to another person.

ABUSE IN OUR SOCIETY

Unfortunately, all forms of abuse—psychological, physical, sexual, material, and neglect—are seen all too often in our society. The number of abuse cases in the United States is rising every day. Some of the ways in which abuse appears in our society are described below.

Criminal Violence

Criminal violence is any violence that breaks a law. This includes stalking; physical abuse such as hitting, pushing, or shoving; and sexual abuse. It's important to note that although emotional and psychological abuse are not considered criminal, they can often lead to criminal violence.

Domestic Violence

Domestic violence occurs if one family member abuses another. It's a serious problem in the United States. Studies estimate that one in four women is a victim of domestic violence.

What's worse, people who abuse their spouses or partners are likely to abuse their children, too.

Child Abuse

Another serious problem in the United States is child abuse. Any harmful behavior or mistreatment of a child is considered **child abuse.**

Warning signs of an abused child include:

- malnutrition
- poor growth pattern
- poor hygiene
- serious dental disorders
- unattended medical needs

If you suspect a child is being abused, you must tell the physician and report it to the authorities. Your responsibility is to report exactly what your suspicions are as well as anything the child has told you. As with all patients, your goal is to meet the health needs of the child. Discuss your suspicions with the physician immediately.

Elder Abuse

Elder abuse is the abuse of an older person. Many older adults depend on others for care. It's estimated that one in ten older adults who depend on others for care is abused or neglected. This kind of abuse may take the form of:

- physical pain or injury
- failure to provide food, water, care, or medication
- involuntary confinement
- withholding sources of income
- sexual abuse
- psychological or emotional abuse

Spousal Abuse

Spousal abuse, the abuse of a spouse or domestic partner, is increasing in the United States. For many spouses, abuse becomes a cycle that seems to have no end. If you suspect a patient is being abused by a spouse, report your suspicion to the physician right away. Most communities have safe places for victims of spousal abuse. The contact information for these places should be part of your office's referral list of community resources.

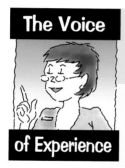

The Voice of Experience

REPORTING PSYCHOLOGICAL OR EMOTIONAL ABUSE IN OLDER ADULT PATIENTS

Q: *One of our office's patients, a 75-year-old woman, has been living with her son and daughter-in-law for the past two years. The patient recently told me that her daughter-in-law verbally abuses her. I've met the patient's daughter-in-law, though, and she seems like a very kind and caring person. I would hate to make an accusation of abuse if it wasn't true. Should I tell the physician anyway?*

A: Any time an older adult patient claims that she is the victim of abuse, it's your legal and ethical duty to report this information to the physician. This holds true even if no other evidence of abuse is present. In addition to a patient's claim of abuse, however, there are several other signs and symptoms of psychological or emotional abuse in older adult patients. Be sure to relate your concerns to the physician if you notice one or more of the following:

- The patient appears to be upset or anxious.
- The patient is extremely withdrawn and does not respond to your questions.
- The patient displays unusual behavior, such as biting or rocking back and forth, with no medical reason for doing so (for example, dementia).

Rape

It's estimated that one out of every eight adult women has been the victim of rape. But it's not unusual for children, adolescents, and even men to be victims of rape. Also, rape is not specific to any socioeconomic or ethnic group. The effects of rape can be devastating to the victim. Many rape victims develop serious mental disorders, as well as drug or alcohol problems as a result of the rape.

Legal Issues and Reporting Requirements

It's important to note that you must consult your office's policy and procedure manual for state and local laws and reporting requirements for criminal violence, domestic violence, elder abuse, child abuse, spousal abuse, and rape.

THERAPEUTIC COMMUNICATION TECHNIQUES

As discussed in other sections of this chapter, you must know which skills and techniques to use in every patient interaction. The situations discussed in this section are especially challenging. The communication skills and techniques you use with patients who are victims of abuse or harassment or who abuse and harass others are critical tools as you work to increase the well-being of the patients in your office.

Suggest Counseling

The abuser and the person who is abused both need help. The physician may encourage these patients to get counseling. Provide information about 24-hour hotlines, support groups, counselors, therapists, and other resources.

Listen to Verbal and Nonverbal Cues

When you suspect that a patient is involved in an abusive situation, listen carefully to the patient's verbal and nonverbal cues. Many patients who are victims of abuse may feel embarrassed or ashamed of their situation. Patients who are abusers may refuse to admit they have a problem. Always remember to observe the body language, facial expressions, and other physical gestures of every patient.

Examine Your Feelings About Abuse

You may find that it's very difficult for you to work with a victim of abuse or with a patient who you suspect is an abuser. Remember that your role is not to judge your patients or their family members or caregivers. Your role is to report any suspicions you have to the physician.

If you feel that your emotions and feelings may prevent you from working effectively with a patient, tell your supervisor. Ask for help or request to be reassigned.

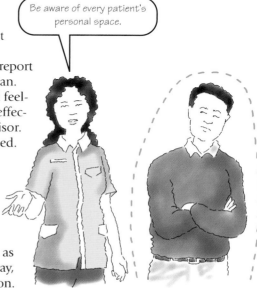

Be aware of every patient's personal space.

Respect Personal Space

A patient who is a victim of abuse may need more personal space than other patients. You should be aware of any nonverbal clues that indicate this need. Look for signs such as the patient's backing away, looking away, or closing his eyes during a conversation.

LEGAL CONSIDERATIONS

The Federal Child Abuse Prevention and Treatment Act states that if you suspect the abuse of a child or older adult, you must report it to the proper authorities. Your identity is protected under this law. In any situation where you suspect abuse, it's also critically important that you write down any information you gather, including exact quotations from the victim. As mentioned before, your office manual should describe the exact procedure to follow when reporting any suspected abuse case.

State-Specific Laws for Reporting Abuse

Each state has different laws for reporting abuse. Patient confidentiality rights do not apply if your state requires you to report certain abusive conditions. Your office's procedure manual should outline the correct procedure to follow when reporting suspected abuse. There is also a national 24-hour hotline at 1-800-4-A-CHILD (1-800-422-4453).

State-Specific Laws for Defining Child Abuse

States differ not only in the way an abuse case is reported, but also in the way child abuse is defined. What is considered a sign of child abuse in one state may not be considered abuse in another state. Check with your office manager or supervisor to find out how your state defines child abuse.

Mandated Reports

You should know to whom you report any suspected abuse case you encounter. In some cases, you're required to report abuse cases to your nurse, physician, or supervisor. In other cases, you report to a risk management representative. Again, consult your office's procedure manual for this information.

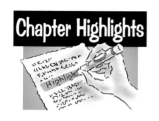

Chapter Highlights

- The medical assistant must be able to communicate effectively with and respond therapeutically to patients with special needs.
- Drug and alcohol addiction is a major health care problem that crosses socioeconomic lines.
- Grief is a reaction that is usually associated with the death of a loved one, but in fact can occur when a person experiences a loss of any kind.
- The medical assistant must be aware of the issues of confidentiality and informed consent when working with patients with HIV or AIDS.

- The medical assistant should offer some suggestions to patients on how to manage stress and anxiety.
- Anger is a natural human emotion that all human beings experience. It can be brought on by fear, threats, or stressful situations.
- The medical assistant should adapt his communication style to meet the needs of individuals with disabilities.
- Each state has laws with specific requirements for reporting abuse.

Active Learning

ROLE PLAYING

Try this role-play activity with one other person. One person is the medical assistant. The other person is an angry patient. Choose two or three situations that might make a patient angry. Work with your partner to identify the verbal and nonverbal communication skills used by the medical assistant in each situation.

Chapter 7

PROVIDING PATIENT WELLNESS AND EDUCATION

Chapter Checklist

- Provide instruction for health maintenance and disease prevention
- Describe the impact of stress on the human body
- Identify coping mechanisms for dealing with stress
- Explain the importance of nutrition and exercise
- Describe the importance of medication and its impact on patient wellness
- Explain general office guidelines that relate to the patient
- Instruct the patient on testing and procedures that occur in the medical office
- Identify community resources for the patient

Chapter Competencies

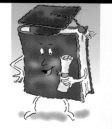

- Orient patients to office policies and procedures (CAAHEP Competency 3.c.3.a. and ABHES Competency 7.a.)
- Instruct individuals according to their needs (CAAHEP Competency 3.c.3.b.)
- Provide instruction for health maintenance and disease prevention (CAAHEP Competency 3.c.3.c. and ABHES Competency 7.c.)
- Identify community resources (CAAHEP Competency 3.c.3.d.)
- Locate resources and information for patients and employers (ABHES Competency 3.f.)

- Schedule and manage appointments (CAAHEP Competency 3.a.1.a. and ABHES Competency 3.c.)
- Apply managed care policies and procedures (CAAHEP Competency 3.a.3.a. and ABHES Competency 3.u.)

A large part of your job as a medical assistant is to help patients learn ways to be and stay healthy. From the moment a patient walks into your office, her experience should be comfortable, supportive, and as positive and stress-free as possible.

In this chapter, you'll learn different ways to educate and instruct patients about living healthfully. You'll explore topics such as stress and its effects on the body, proper nutrition, and the benefits of exercise. You'll learn how to teach patients important information about their medications. You'll also learn how to explain general office policies that relate to the patient.

Promoting Health Maintenance and Disease Prevention

One of the most important skills you learn as a medical assistant is how to teach patients about their health and medical conditions. Teaching patients how to lead healthy lifestyles is often the first step to health maintenance. **Health maintenance** involves preventing diseases and staying as healthy as possible at all times. Working with patients to help them understand how to be healthy is a rewarding and fulfilling part of the medical assistant's job.

STYLES OF LEARNING

As a medical assistant, you'll provide education for many different types of learners from many different age groups. Each patient will have his own unique learning style. Patients can learn from the cognitive, affective, or psychomotor domains. Visual (sight) learners, auditory (hearing) learners, and tactile (touch) learners are three different types of learners. Each of these types requires a different teaching approach. It's important for you to be able to adapt your teaching style and educational tools and materials to accommodate the learning styles and needs of your patients.

KNOWLEDGE IS KEY

It's important for you to teach patients about their health. When you educate patients, you help them find the answers to questions about their health. You also provide support and inspire them to lead healthy lives.

PATIENT EDUCATION AND TEACHING

As a medical assistant, you help and teach patients in many ways. This may be as simple as reminding a patient how often to take a certain medication. Or it could be as challenging as helping a patient through a grieving process. Whatever the task may be, excellent communication skills help ensure your success. You can also use the communication skills you've learned to teach patients about health and wellness.

The ways you listen, send messages, and give feedback are some of the key communication skills you use with patients. In addition, use the skills described in the sections that follow to educate and teach patients effectively.

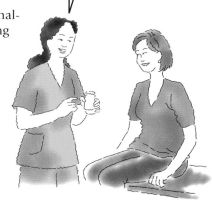

Remember, Mrs. Green, the physician said you should take one tablet every four hours until all the tablets are gone.

Stay Current

It seems like there is always something new in the medical field. Take time to stay informed about current trends, discoveries, and issues in medicine. You can do this easily by becoming a member of a professional organization, reading medical and science magazines, or by checking the Internet for medical news. Having the latest knowledge about medical issues will help you communicate effectively with patients.

Know Your Community's Resources

Know what your community has to offer patients. Support groups, special organizations, and other community organizations can provide valuable services. If possible, speak to the contact people for the major organizations and support groups in your community. Find out as much as you can about what services are offered, when meetings take place, and what kinds of activities are scheduled throughout the year. Be prepared to provide information on community resources to patients.

Use Teaching Tools

Using preprinted handouts, models, charts, DVDs, or other teaching tools is a good way to help educate patients. Models, charts, and DVDs can be used in the office to further explain a patient's diagnosis or treatment plan. Patients can take handouts home with them and look over the information at their own convenience. Have brochures and information sheets available and provide a list of reliable websites where patients can go for additional information. If you do not have the information a patient needs, tell the patient you'll get back to him as soon as you can get it.

Allow a Time and Place for Teaching

When you need to teach or instruct a patient about a specific topic, make sure you have set aside a quiet room and have given yourself enough time. You do not want a lack of time or distractions to interfere with your instructions.

Provide Written Instructions

It can be helpful to provide information or instructions in written form. This gives patients something they can refer to after they leave the office. Always make sure the office phone number is included with written information, so that patients can call if they have questions.

Encourage Questions

Always encourage patients to ask questions. Patients often do not have questions until after they have left your office. Provide patients with the office phone number and remind them that they can call with any questions they think of after they go home.

Ask for Feedback

After you have spent time instructing or explaining something, ask questions to make sure the patient understands. If you sense that the patient does not understand, present your information in a different way—maybe by writing out the key points.

Document All Patient Education

Remember to document all teachings that have occurred in the patient's medical record. Documentation should include the following:

- date and time of teaching
- what information was taught
- how the information was taught

- evaluation of teaching (how well the patient is able to adapt or apply the new information)
- any additional teaching planned

DATE	TIME	ORDERS
11/13/XX	9:35 AM	*Patient arrived in the office for teaching on the glucose meter; brought meter from home. Following steps were demonstrated by me: calibration of meter strips, battery change, finger sticks, strip insertion into machine, use of the patient logbook. Normal blood glucose ranges were reviewed along with the treatment of low blood sugar. Pt. returned demonstration without problem. Reviewed glucose meter instruction manual with pt. Pt. instructed to bring logbook to each MD appointment.*
		— M. Garcia, CMA

Proper documentation is important because from a legal viewpoint, procedures are only considered to have been done if they are recorded.

MAINTAINING HEALTHY LIFESTYLES

Of course, one of your main goals as a medical assistant is to teach patients how to live healthfully. However, it's also important for you to maintain a healthy lifestyle as well. In this section, you'll explore in detail five key factors that contribute to health maintenance. These factors are:

- reducing stress
- getting proper nutrition
- exercising regularly
- getting enough rest
- taking medications correctly

Reduce Stress

Learning what stress is and how to cope with stress is a key to leading a healthy lifestyle. **Stress** is the mind and body's response or reaction to a real or imagined threat, event, or change. You should be aware of the things in your life that cause negative stress. By becoming aware of these things, you can then find ways to reduce unwanted stress in your life. For example, you might discover that Wednesdays are especially stressful days at work. To help reduce this stress, schedule something enjoyable for Wednesday evening, such as a hot bubble bath, a workout at the local gym, a brisk walk with a friend, or a few hours of reading your favorite novel. Encourage patients to reduce stress in their lives as part of their own health maintenance plans.

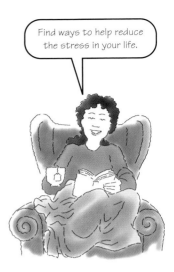

Find ways to help reduce the stress in your life.

Get Proper Nutrition

Learning how to eat healthfully every day is a skill that often takes practice. Using the Food Guide Pyramid to plan meals and snacks helps make this task easier. Teach patients what the Food Guide Pyramid means and how they can use it.

Exercise Regularly

Regular exercise is one of the most healthful habits anyone can have. Helping patients see and experience the benefits of exercise is a big part of teaching patients about a healthy lifestyle.

Get Enough Rest

All bodies need to rest. When you sleep or rest, your body renews and repairs itself. Also, a rested body is better able to deal with stress. Encourage patients to get enough rest every day.

Take Medications as Prescribed

Medications are prescribed to help prevent, cure, or manage certain medical or health problems. But medications can do their job only if they are taken correctly as prescribed. Make sure patients understand how to take their medications properly.

Stress

On a typical day, you might wake up, go to work, do your job, come home, spend time with family and friends, and go to bed. You go through your normal routine without really being aware of it. But when stress happens, it can change your normal routine. The change could be big or small, positive or negative, challenging or threatening. The change could be related to work or to personal life. Stress happens frequently, so the ability for you and your patients to respond to it in a healthy way is critical.

IMPACT ON THE BODY

When stress occurs, it can affect every part of a person's being—physical, intellectual, social, spiritual, and emotional. And since every person is different, one individual's response to stress may be completely different from another individual's response to the same stress.

You may get stressed out when there is a lot of traffic on the road. As a result of this stress, you may get a pounding headache. Another person may respond to traffic by becoming very angry. Yet another person may get a stomachache. Everyone's body responds differently to stress.

Causes of Stress

The cause of stress is called a **stressor.** Stressors can be internal factors such as illness, fear, and chemical changes within the body. Stressors can also be external factors such as loss, tragedy, and loud noises. For example, an internal stressor might be a pulled muscle, a fear of spiders, or a hormone change that causes depression. An external stressor might be the loss of a loved one, a serious accident, or constant noise from construction.

Types of Stress

As you have read, stressors are threats, events, or changes that cause stress. A stressor is neither positive nor negative. Stress, however, can be positive or negative. Positive stress and negative stress can happen together or separately, and the same stressor can cause positive stress for some people, but negative stress for others.

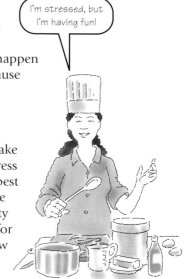

I'm stressed, but I'm having fun!

Positive Stress

Positive stress is stress that is motivating. It can make a person energized, creative, and aware. Positive stress can help a person work better and perform to the best of her abilities. Challenges tend to produce positive stress. New responsibilities at work, the opportunity to give a speech at a family gathering, performing for an audience, or something as simple as trying a new recipe can cause positive stress. Positive stress can cause good changes in a person's life.

Negative Stress

Negative stress is stress that makes a person tense, anxious, angry, or depressed. Fearful events, threats, and tragedies are examples of things that can produce negative stress. People usually work less efficiently when they are negatively stressed.

COPING MECHANISMS

Remember that what produces positive stress in one person may produce negative stress in another. For example, people respond in different ways to the idea of performing in front of an audience. Some people shake nervously, become sick to their stomach, sweat, and get headaches at the thought of being on a stage. Other people become inspired and invigorated when they prepare to perform.

People can use different coping mechanisms to handle stress. A **coping mechanism** is a way of lessening the negative effects of stress or a stressor. Some coping mechanisms are listed below. Each one will be described separately in this section. You can tell patients about these coping mechanisms to help them reduce and manage the stress in their lives.

- Avoid stressors.
- Limit your number of activities.
- Talk to someone.
- Exercise regularly.
- Get proper nutrition.
- Redirect negative energy.
- Relax.

Avoid Stressors

Of course, the most logical way to prevent a particular kind of stress is to avoid the stressor that causes it. However, this might not always be possible. If you need to, you can limit stress that is caused by performing in front of an audience by avoiding situations that require performing. But you can't avoid stress that is caused by events and situations that are out of your control. For instance, delayed flights at the airport may be a stressor. This stressor is difficult to avoid if you need to fly on a particular day. If you can't avoid a stressor, try another coping mechanism.

Limit Activities

A common stressor is feeling overwhelmed by having to do too much at once. People can avoid this stressor by learning to prioritize their responsibilities and activities. Do not be afraid to say "no" when someone asks you to volunteer for an activity or event. If you feel the need to stay at home and rest, cancel your date to go shopping. Remember the importance of rest and relaxation, and plan your activities accordingly.

Trying to do too much at once causes stress.

Talk to Someone

One of the most enjoyable ways to deal with stress is by talking to a friend. Sometimes, just the act of describing stressors and stressful situations to a caring friend works wonders. In fact, a person might feel instantly better by just saying the words, "I'm so stressed out!"

Exercise

Exercise is a great way to cope with stress. There are many ways to exercise. The trick is finding an enjoyable way to exercise regularly. You should look forward to exercise. You should feel invigorated while you're exercising, as well as when you're finished exercising. Here are some examples of isotonic, isometric, and isokinetic exercises:

- *Isotonic.* Isotonic exercise involves muscle shortening and active movement. Examples include running, jogging, walking, bicycling, swimming, and tennis.
- *Isometric.* Isometric exercise involves muscle contraction but no shortening and no active movement. Examples include tensing and relaxing muscles groups in the thigh, abdomen, calf, or arm.
- *Isokinetic.* Isokinetic exercise involves muscle contraction and some active movement. Examples include lifting weights and range-of-motion exercises.

Redirect Negative Energy

Another way to cope with stress is to redirect the energy created by negative stress. Instead of letting the energy come out as nervousness or anxiety, use it to accomplish something useful. Some ways to redirect nervous energy include:

- cleaning the kitchen
- vacuuming
- writing in a journal

- composing a poem
- singing
- playing a musical instrument
- painting or drawing a picture
- cooking a special meal for somebody
- making a gift for a friend

Get Proper Nutrition

Eating a balanced diet and drinking plenty of water make it easier for the body to cope with stress when it happens. Making healthy food choices, moderating caffeine intake, and not skipping meals help the body fight the effects of negative stress. The next section will discuss the importance of nutrition in more detail.

Relax

Learning to relax and stay calm makes it much easier to handle stress when it happens. Relaxation is also important after a stressful situation has passed. Responding to stress requires energy. Depending on the seriousness of the stress, the body can become very tired and fatigued. For this reason, once a stressful situation has passed, you should allow your body to rest and relax.

Listen to This **COPING WITH STRESS**
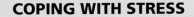
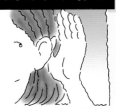

Try these helpful ways to cope with the stressors in your life and recommend them to patients.

- When you recognize that you're feeling anxious, call or visit a friend. A trusted friend will be glad to let you "blow off some steam" by listening to your problems.
- Sometimes, stress is caused when you try to do things perfectly. Remind yourself that trying to be perfect or do things perfectly is a battle that you can't win. Learn to accept some imperfections. Imperfections are a part of what makes you different from everybody else!
- Make a list of your daily, weekly, and monthly responsibilities. If you're doing too much, think about the activities you can cut back or eliminate.

RELAXATION TECHNIQUES

Learning how to relax may be the biggest key to helping reduce stress. There are many ways to relax. It's important that each person find the relaxation technique that is best for her.

Breathing Techniques

The best thing about using breathing techniques to relax is that these techniques can be done anywhere and at any time. The body requires large amounts of oxygen to do all it has to do. It's easy to get into the habit of breathing shallowly and inefficiently. Breathing deeply and efficiently brings in more oxygen and gets rid of more carbon dioxide with each breath. Try this simple breathing exercise:

1. Sit straight up on a chair.
2. Place your hands on your stomach.
3. Take a deep breath in through your nose.
4. Feel your hands being pushed away by your stomach.
5. Hold the breath for a few seconds.
6. Exhale through your mouth.
7. Feel your hands being pulled in toward your stomach.

Visualization

Visualization is a relaxation technique in which people allow their minds to wander and imagine freely. During visualization, people focus on positive images, ideas, and situations. For example, you might visualize yourself floating through the air like a bird, lying in a field of grass, or sleeping on a tropical beach.

Physical Exercise

Physical exercise is an excellent coping mechanism for stress. Regular physical exercise not only helps reduce stress but also increases a person's ability to relax, helps reduce tension, and keeps the heart and circulatory system healthy. You'll read more about exercise later in this chapter.

Exercise helps reduce stress.

Nutrition

What people eat plays a large role in their overall health. The food choices you make every day affect the way your body is able to function. It's not hard to eat a healthy diet. Some basic information, common sense, and a trip to the grocery store are the only tools you need!

WHAT IS NUTRITION?

Nutrition is the science of food and how different foods affect a person's health. Every kind of food that you take into your body is broken down into smaller parts. The cells in your body use these small food parts to keep your body running smoothly.

BASIC FACTS TO TEACH PATIENTS

Many people try to lose weight to get healthy. But cutting out important foods from their diets is not the best way to do this. Teaching patients some basic facts about good nutrition can help them be healthier. The following list includes tips for healthy eating and weight loss that you can pass on to patients.

- Eat a balanced diet; this is the key to good nutrition.
- Never cut entire food groups from your diet to lose weight.
- Include a combination of colors—red apples, orange carrots, green peppers—in each meal.
- Limit your salt and sodium intake.
- Eat three balanced meals per day.
- Avoid eating at least two hours before going to bed.
- Drink plenty of water.
- Limit your fat intake.
- Avoid drinking too much soda and beverages with caffeine.

THE FOOD GUIDE PYRAMID

The U.S. Department of Agriculture (USDA) suggests using a tool called the Food Guide Pyramid to help you plan what to eat each day. This is a handy way to figure out which foods you need more or less of. You can access the Food Guide Pyramid through the Internet at www.mypyramid.gov. You might want to have handouts of the Food Guide Pyramid available for patients. If patients are unfamiliar with the Food Guide Pyramid, teach them how to use it.

Pyramid Sections

The Food Guide Pyramid is divided into six sections—one section for each of the five main food groups and one section for oils and fats. The foods that you should eat more of take up a larger slice of the Food Guide Pyramid. The foods you should eat sparingly take up the smallest slice of the pyramid.

Grains

The largest section of the pyramid is the food group that includes breads, cereals, grains, and pasta. It's recommended that you eat 6 to 11 servings from this group each day. If possible, try to eat more whole grain foods, which contain more nutrients. A typical serving size from this food group could be:

- 1 slice of whole grain bread
- ½ cup of cooked rice, pasta, or cereal
- 1 ounce of ready-to-eat cereal
- ½ English muffin

Vegetables

The next two largest sections after the grains group are the vegetable group and the fruit group. You should eat three to five servings from the vegetable group each day. A typical serving from the vegetable group could be:

- ½ cup of chopped raw or cooked vegetables
- 1 cup of leafy green raw vegetables

Fruits

You should eat two to four servings from the fruit group each day. A typical serving from this group could be:

- 1 medium piece of fruit or melon wedge
- ¾ cup of juice
- ½ cup of canned fruit
- ¼ cup of dried fruit

Milk

After the vegetable and fruit groups are two more sections—the milk group and the meat and beans group. The milk group includes milk, yogurt, cheese, cottage cheese, and other dairy products. The USDA suggests that you eat two to three servings from this group each day. A typical serving might be:

- 1 cup of skim or low-fat milk or yogurt
- 1½ ounces of natural cheese
- 2 ounces of processed cheese

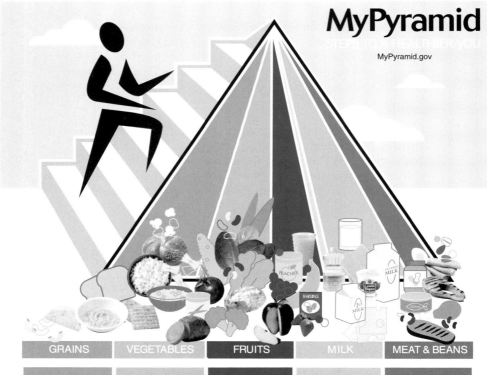

MyPyramid

STEPS TO A HEALTHIER YOU

MyPyramid.gov

GRAINS	VEGETABLES	FRUITS	MILK	MEAT & BEANS
GRAINS Make half your grains whole	**VEGETABLES** Vary your veggies	**FRUITS** Focus on fruits	**MILK** Get your calcium-rich foods	**MEAT & BEANS** Go lean with protein
Eat at least 3 oz. of whole-grain cereals, breads, crackers, rice, or pasta every day 1 oz. is about 1 slice of bread, about 1 cup of breakfast cereal, or ½ cup of cooked rice, cereal, or pasta	Eat more dark-green veggies like broccoli, spinach, and other dark leafy greens Eat more orange vegetables like carrots and sweetpotatoes Eat more dry beans and peas like pinto beans, kidney beans, and lentils	Eat a variety of fruit Choose fresh, frozen, canned, or dried fruit Go easy on fruit juices	Go low-fat or fat-free when you choose milk, yogurt, and other milk products If you don't or can't consume milk, choose lactose-free products or other calcium sources such as fortified foods and beverages	Choose low-fat or lean meats and poultry Bake it, broil it, or grill it Vary your protein routine — choose more fish, beans, peas, nuts, and seeds

For a 2,000-calorie diet, you need the amounts below from each food group. To find the amounts that are right for you, go to MyPyramid.gov.

Eat 6 oz. every day	Eat 2½ cups every day	Eat 2 cups every day	Get 3 cups every day; for kids aged 2 to 8, it's 2	Eat 5½ oz. every day

Find your balance between food and physical activity

Be sure to stay within your daily calorie needs.

Be physically active for at least 30 minutes most days of the week.

About 60 minutes a day of physical activity may be needed to prevent weight gain.

For sustaining weight loss, at least 60 to 90 minutes a day of physical activity may be required.

Children and teenagers should be physically active for 60 minutes every day, or most days.

Know the limits on fats, sugars, and salt (sodium)

Make most of your fat sources from fish, nuts, and vegetable oils.

Limit solid fats like butter, stick margarine, shortening, and lard, as well as foods that contain these.

Check the Nutrition Facts label to keep saturated fats, trans fats, and sodium low.

Choose food and beverages low in added sugars. Added sugars contribute calories with few, if any, nutrients.

MyPyramid.gov
STEPS TO A HEALTHIER YOU

U.S. Department of Agriculture
Center for Nutrition Policy and Promotion
April 2005
CNPP-15

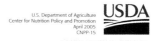

USDA

Meat and Beans

This group is made up of foods that are high in protein. It's recommended that you eat two to three servings from this food group. A typical serving could be:

- 2½ to 3 ounces of cooked lean meat, poultry, or fish
- 1 ounce of lean meat = ½ cup of cooked beans, 1 egg, or 2 tablespoons of peanut butter

Oils

The smallest sliver of the Food Guide Pyramid, and the food group that should make up the least amount of what you eat, is the oils group. These are foods such as shortening, olive oil, many salad dressings, and butter.

Teaching Tips

Here are some tips you can teach patients about choosing foods and planning meals.

- Eat darker breads and avoid white bread, croissants, biscuits, and pastries.
- Choose cereals that are oat, bran, and whole grain.
- Buy fruits that are fresh, frozen, dried, and canned (in water or juice) so that you always have a supply on hand.
- Eat vegetables without butter or sauces.
- Choose low-fat cheese, skim or 1% milk, and 1% or 2% cottage cheese.
- Look for the freshest fish.
- Limit the amount of bacon you eat or cook with or select turkey bacon instead.
- Choose USDA-select grade beef.
- Choose low-fat snacks such as air-popped popcorn, pretzels, and rice cakes.

DIETARY GUIDELINES

The USDA and U.S. Department of Health and Human Services have developed guidelines to help improve people's diets. These guidelines should be used along with the Food Guide Pyramid to help choose and plan meals wisely.

Nutrition Facts Labels

Food products include labels that describe the nutritional content of the food. Knowing how to read and interpret these labels is key to making healthy food choices. There is a lot of

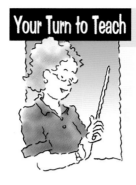

Your Turn to Teach

USING THE FOOD GUIDE PYRAMID

Patients might think that using the Food Guide Pyramid is too confusing or difficult. It's really easier than it seems! Help patients get used to using the pyramid and practicing good nutrition by sharing the following tips:

- Choose a variety of foods from each of the food groups on the pyramid. Not only does this help you eat a balanced diet, it makes eating more interesting!

> The Food Guide Pyramid makes it easy to substitute foods.

- Use the pyramid along with your own tastes and preferences. Do not think that a serving from the bread and cereal group can only be a slice of bread or a half cup of cooked cereal. You could also have wild rice, pasta, grits, bulgur wheat, cornmeal, or popcorn.

- Combine foods from each food group. A quesadilla could include a hot corn tortilla, melted cheddar cheese, and some grilled chicken pieces. Add some chopped tomatoes and greens, and you have a deliciously balanced meal!

- Always aim for nutrient-rich foods. Choose wisely when selecting foods. Substitute foods if necessary. For example, if you're lactose intolerant, use foods from the meat and beans group in place of those from the milk group.

nutritional information on food labels! The nutrition facts label for a food product lists the amount of saturated fat, cholesterol, sodium, dietary fiber, sugars, protein, vitamins, minerals, and calories per serving of that food item. Teach patients how to read and understand these labels so they can make good food choices.

Serving Size

The Food Guide Pyramid recommends a certain number of servings per day from each food group. Remember that the number of servings does *not* mean the number of bananas, or hamburgers, or slices of bread, or cups of pasta you should have each day. For example, one serving of pasta is a half cup. A typical dinner size helping of spaghetti might be one to two cups of pasta. This is actually two to four servings. Also keep in mind that one serving of fresh fruit refers to a medium-sized piece of fruit. Many fruits, like apples, bananas, and pears, come in different sizes. A large banana could be equal to two servings.

Help patients understand serving sizes by describing many examples. You may wish to show them different measuring cups. You may also wish to show examples of serving sizes with pictures or models.

> Compare a serving size of meat to something patients are familiar with, such as a deck of playing cards, so they can serve themselves a healthful portion of meat at meals.

Healthy Food Preparation

There are also healthy ways to prepare food. Following these food preparation tips will help you keep your servings from the oils group to a minimum. Share these healthy food preparation tips with patients.

- Trim fat off beef. Use a cooking rack so that fat can drip off the meat during cooking.
- Broil, boil, bake, roast, or grill instead of frying.
- Remove skin from chicken. Always wash your hands and cutting surfaces after preparing chicken.
- Skim fat from homemade soups.
- Use unsaturated oils (canola, safflower, corn) instead of saturated fats (lard, butter).
- Use nonstick sprays when possible.

SPECIAL DIETS

Sometimes a patient's medical condition or situation will require diet restrictions and special foods. Some chronic conditions such as diabetes and heart disease require special diets. When the physician orders such a diet for a patient, you may be responsible for teaching the patient how to follow the guidelines.

Exercise

By now you know that exercise is important for good health. It's also important to choose a type of exercise that you enjoy doing and that gives you the benefits you need most. Or, you might choose a variety of exercises to include in your personal fitness plan. The physician may recommend specific exercises to a patient. This section will discuss the benefits of exercise and explain the differences between active and passive exercise.

HOW IS EXERCISE DEFINED?

Exercise is any activity that uses muscles voluntarily or involuntarily to help maintain fitness. There are exercises you can do sitting in a chair or standing in line at the grocery store. You do not have to wear special clothes to exercise. You can exercise in old sweats, work clothes, or your pajamas. One of the most critical parts of doing any exercise is that you do it regularly. It's important to explain the benefits of exercise to patients. Knowing and understanding the benefits of exercise can give them the incentive they need to keep up a regular exercise routine.

Moderate exercise has many health benefits.

BENEFITS TO THE BODY

For some people, the hardest part of any exercise routine is starting. Sometimes, patients are so overwhelmed by the idea of spending hours a day lifting weights and running that they never give exercise a chance. If a patient seems hesitant to start an exercise routine, you may want to remind her that any exercise, even 5 minutes a day, is better than none at all. From 5 minutes a day, a person can gradually add a couple of minutes here or there until she is exercising for 10, 20, or 30 minutes a day. Even a moderate exercise routine has many health benefits, such as reducing stress, maintaining a healthy body weight, and increasing circulation and muscle tone.

Reduces Stress

When you're stressed for long periods of time, your body gets tired. It takes energy for your body to deal with stress. Even though it takes energy to exercise, the body gets energized when it exercises. After an exercise routine, a person may feel refreshed and rejuvenated. Exercise helps reduce stress and helps a person deal with stressors better.

Maintains Healthy Body Weight

It takes energy to exercise. Where does this energy come from? One way the body gets energy is from body fat. The cells that make up body fat have a lot of stored energy in them. Regular exercise uses some of this fat for energy. As excess fat is used up, the body becomes trimmer.

Increases Circulation

What's the first thing you notice when you start exercising? It's probably your heart rate. When you lift more, move faster, or kick higher, your body responds by moving blood faster. The more people do, the more energy their body cells need. Body cells work harder during exercise. When cells work harder, they need more fuel to make more energy. This fuel includes things like glucose, oxygen, and other nutrients. Nutrients are carried in the blood to each cell by the circulatory system. Every beat of the heart moves blood and nutrients to every cell in the body. And the harder and faster the heart beats, the faster the nutrients get to the cells. So, when people exercise, their circulation increases.

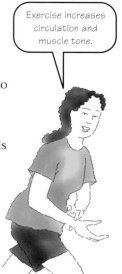

Exercise increases circulation and muscle tone.

Increases Muscle Tone

Another benefit of exercise is increased muscle tone. Muscle cells function by contracting and relaxing. Muscle cells in your leg may help you kick a soccer ball. Muscle cells in your heart keep blood pumping throughout your life. When muscles contract and relax efficiently, they are toned. The movements and increased circulation of exercise help keep your muscles fit.

TYPES OF EXERCISE

Earlier in this chapter, you read about three kinds of exercise: isotonic, isometric, and isokinetic. But another way to classify exercise is by dividing it into two groups: active exercise and passive exercise.

Active Exercise

In **active exercise,** people move their bodies by themselves. Active exercise improves joint mobility and increases muscle mass, muscle tone, strength, and circulation in the body parts being exercised. Examples of active exercise include running, swimming, walking, and jogging.

Passive Exercise

When people are unable to move their bodies by themselves, they can participate in passive exercise. In **passive exercise,** a therapist, nurse, or caregiver helps a person move each joint through its range of motion (ROM). ROM exercises keep joints healthy and mobile. They also keep circulation in the joints strong.

Both active and passive exercises keep joints moving and increase circulation to the joints being exercised. However, only active exercise has the added benefit of improving cardiac and respiratory function.

PHYSICIAN CONSULTATION AND CLEARANCE

If patients are over the age of 35, they should see their physician before starting an exercise routine. If a patient is pregnant, she should check with her physician before starting an exercise program.

If a patient can't move his body to do active exercise, he can do passive ROM exercises with the help of a family member or friend. The family member or friend should seek training from a therapist or physician before helping with the ROM exercises.

Medications

Medications are given to a patient in the form of a prescription. This order is written by a physician or, in some cases, a nurse practitioner. A medication is ordered for a specific reason. It's important that patients take any medication exactly as the physician instructs. Part of your job is to make sure that patients understand the physician's instructions for taking medications.

PHARMACEUTICAL INFORMATION SHEETS

Important information about a medication is listed on a pharmaceutical information sheet. This sheet accompanies the medication when a patient picks it up at a pharmacy. Encourage patients to read the pharmaceutical information sheets every time they fill a new prescription. Tell patients that if they have any questions, they should ask their pharmacist or call the physician.

TEACHING PATIENTS ABOUT MEDICATIONS

Taking medication can be confusing. Make sure you go over all prescriptions with patients. Get feedback to make sure patients understand when they should take the medication, how much they should take, and how long they should take it for. Talk with patients about issues related to the medication such as dosage, route of administration, purpose, use, side effects, changes in body function, activities to avoid, and other drug interactions. Each of these issues is discussed in more detail below.

Medication Name

The prescription provided by the physician includes the name of the drug. This can be a brand name or a generic name. In some cases, the physician may prefer that the patient use a brand name medication. Many medication names are long and difficult to pronounce. Write out the name of the medication to help patients remember it.

Dosage

The dosage is how much, how often, and for how long a patient needs to take a medication. It might be helpful to write down each day's dosage for a patient on a calendar. This way, the patient can easily check when to start taking the medication, when to stop, and how much to take each day.

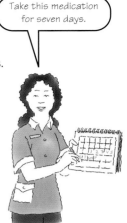

Take this medication for seven days.

Route of Administration

Medications can be administered to the body in different ways. The way a medication is taken is called the *route of administration.* It's important that the prescription state the route of administration. Routes for administering medication include:

- by mouth (oral)
- under the tongue (sublingual)
- between the cheek and gum (buccal)
- by inserting into the vagina (vaginal)
- by inserting into the rectum (rectal)
- by applying to the skin (topical, transdermal)
- by injection (intradermal, intramuscular, subcutaneous)
- into a vein (intravenous)

Purpose

A patient should know why he is taking a medication. Make sure you explain the purpose of a medication to a patient. Also explain how soon the patient should expect to see a result from taking a medication. You may recommend to patients that they keep a list of their medications, including correct dosages and the reason each medication has been prescribed.

Use

Some medications are prescribed to be taken every day for an indefinite period of time. Other medications are prescribed for a brief time. The physician may prescribe a medication to use only when a patient has certain symptoms such as nausea, joint pain, headache, or inability to sleep. If a patient has injured himself, he may have been prescribed a medication for pain or an antibiotic to help his body fight off infection.

It's important that patients know when and for how long they should use a certain medication. Tell patients that they should call the physician's office if they have any questions about their medication.

Possible Side Effects

Almost all medications produce some side effects. A side effect may be minor, such as a brief bout of nausea, a slight headache, or a feeling of dizziness or drowsiness. These kinds of side effects are usually not serious and may go unnoticed.

However, some side effects are serious. You should make patients aware of all potential side effects of a medication. Let patients know that they should call the physician immediately if they experience a serious side effect. Serious side effects include:

- bleeding from the rectum
- blood in the urine
- unconsciousness
- rash
- fever
- diarrhea
- vomiting

Changes in Body Functions

Make patients aware that some medications may affect certain body organs or organ systems. As a result, patients may notice changes in their:

- urine
- feces
- breath
- skin color
- whites of eyes
- skin texture
- body odor
- digestion
- ability to concentrate
- ability to sleep
- coordination

If a patient notices a change that concerns her, she should call her physician.

Possible Interactions

Some medications should not be taken at the same time as other medications. This is because the action of one medication may conflict with the action of another. The combination of certain medications can also make a person sick. To prevent this from happening, make sure the physician knows about all medications, vitamins, supplements, and herbal remedies that a patient is taking.

Activities to Avoid

The side effects of some medications may make it difficult to perform certain activities. For example, some medications may make a person drowsy or sleepy. People should not drive vehicles when taking such medications. They should also avoid activities that require them to be alert and focused.

Every medication comes with special stickers that caution the patient about what to avoid while taking the medication. Encourage patients to pay close attention to these stickers.

MEDICATION THERAPY TEACHING TOOL

Teaching patients about medication is important to help them take responsibility for their own health. Patients should understand and be aware of the purpose and dosage of any medicine

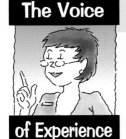

The Voice of Experience

MEDICATION TIPS

Q: *What are some ways I can help patients keep their medications organized?*

A: It's easy for patients who take several medications to get them confused. Here are some handy tips you can share with patients to help them keep their medications up to date and organized:

- Go through all medications monthly (maybe on the first day of each month) and throw out any that are outdated.
- Store medications where children and pets can't get to them.
- Make a list of all medications and dosages. Post this list on the refrigerator. Keep a copy of this list in your wallet or purse for emergencies and visits to the physician.
- Remind patients not to memorize a medication based on the color or shape of the tablet, capsule, or pill. Different companies make the same medication in different colors and shapes. Encourage patients to memorize the name and dose of each medication.
- Use a weekly pill dispenser (available at grocery and drug stores) to prepare the entire week's worth of medication.
- Mark on a calendar when a medication needs to be refilled.

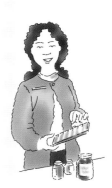

they are taking. Preparing a medication therapy teaching tool for your patients will help them understand their medications. A medication therapy teaching tool should include the following information:

- medication name (generic or brand name)
- dosage
- route of administration
- purpose of the medication
- possible changes in body functions
- possible side effects
- other medications (including over-the-counter medicines and supplements) that might interfere with the action of the medication
- foods or liquids to be avoided
- activities to be avoided
- phone number to call for any questions or concerns

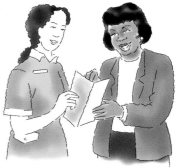

Prepare a medication therapy teaching tool to help patients understand their medication.

For commonly prescribed medications, it's helpful to keep preprinted medication therapy teaching tools on hand.

Understanding Office Procedures

Your office has certain procedures that you must be familiar with. Missed appointments, schedule changes, walk-ins, cancellations, and other situations should be handled smoothly and efficiently according to the policies of your medical office. Because every office is different, it's important that patients are made aware of how such procedures are handled at your office.

EXPLAINING OFFICE GUIDELINES

The guidelines and policies at your office may be quite different from the medical office a new patient has come from. One of your tasks as a medical assistant is to make sure every patient is aware of the policies at your office. In some cases, certain policies can be posted in writing. In other cases, you may have to inform a patient verbally about specific guidelines or rules.

Appointment Reminders

There are a number of ways to let patients know about their next scheduled appointment. A patient reminder tells a patient when he should make his next appointment, or when his next appointment is scheduled. This reminder can be an appointment card with the information written on it. The card can be given or mailed to the patient. A reminder can also be a phone call to a patient or an e-mail reminder.

An appointment card is usually given to the patient as she leaves the office. The card should have the following information on it:

- patient's name
- day, date, and time of the next appointment
- physician's name and phone number

It's important to give the patient an appointment card only for her next appointment. Even though some patients have scheduled a series of appointments, it's less confusing for the patient to give her an appointment card for one appointment at a time.

Another way to help remind patients of an appointment is by phone. This can be as simple as saying, "Hello, Mr. Palmer. This is Libby from Dr. Reed's office. I'm calling to confirm your appointment for tomorrow, Thursday, February 10, at 3:30 P.M." Unless the patient has questions for you, you can simply say, "Thank you. See you then!" and hang up. Be sure to note on a list the patients who have been given phone reminders. This helps prevent patients from getting multiple phone reminders.

Mailed or e-mailed reminders may be used by your office as a general procedure for all patients. They may also be used for patients who do not wish to receive phone reminders or who could not be reached by phone. These reminders should be sent at least a week before the scheduled appointment. A mailed or e-mailed reminder can also be used to let a patient know about the need for a specific annual procedure such as a Pap smear, mammogram, or prostate examination. Having preprinted cards on hand makes filling out mailed reminders easier. Many offices send mailed reminder cards in envelopes to protect patient privacy.

Medical Emergencies

Occasionally, a patient calls or comes into the office who needs to be seen right away. A patient experiencing a medical emergency will have to be worked into an existing schedule. Usually, in this kind of situation, other patients are willing to reschedule their appointments. Your office may have specific policies on how patients should handle a medical emergency. Make patients aware of these policies verbally and in writing.

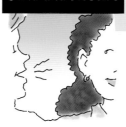

Send and Receive

SCHEDULE CHANGES FOR PATIENT EMERGENCIES

Suppose a patient walks into the office with a medical emergency. The schedule is already booked for the day, and the waiting room is nearly full. What do you do? Here are some ineffective and effective ways to handle this situation.

Mr. Choi walks into the office with his right hand bandaged. He explains to the receptionist that he cut his hand while slicing vegetables and can't stop the bleeding. He asks to see the physician immediately.

Ineffective:

- The receptionist greets Mr. Choi by saying, "Hello, sir. Do you have an appointment?"
- Mr. Choi, cradling his hand, says, "No, I just cut my hand, and I think I need to see Dr. Beech right away."
- "Well, as you can see, Mr. Choi, we are very busy today. I'll see if Dr. Beech can work you in. Have a seat, and I'll let you know."

When a patient who has just suffered an injury walks into the office, it's important to immediately determine whether the patient is experiencing a medical emergency. If the patient's wound or injury is bleeding uncontrollably or if the wound is large and open, the patient must see a physician immediately. If the patient seems frantic or if it seems like the patient may go into shock, it's important to get him into an examination room right away.

Effective:

- The receptionist sees that Mr. Choi has a bandaged hand and immediately says, "Have you just injured yourself?"
- Mr. Choi replies, "Yes, I was slicing vegetables and I cut my hand. My hand is bleeding a lot."
- The receptionist gets additional information from the patient by asking a few questions, "Can you tell me how and when the accident happened? Is this the same bandage that you put on the wound when the accident occurred?"

- Mr. Choi is anxious and has to think hard to answer these questions. His color is a little pale. The receptionist calls a nurse immediately to take Mr. Choi into an examination room.

In this situation, it may also be necessary to reschedule one or more of the patients with regularly scheduled appointments. Medical emergencies happen. Learning how to handle them smoothly and efficiently is a skill required by all who work in a medical office.

Walk-in Patients

Suppose a patient comes to the office without a scheduled appointment and expects to see the physician. As mentioned before, a walk-in patient with a medical emergency must be seen right away. Your office may have special policies for dealing with other walk-in patients. You may ask the patient to take a seat in the waiting room. Then you can ask the patient's physician to decide whether to see the patient. If the physician decides to see the patient, try to work her in as easily as possible. Politely remind the patient of the office's appointment scheduling policy to ensure that she schedules her appointment the next time. If the physician decides not to see the patient, ask the patient to schedule an appointment.

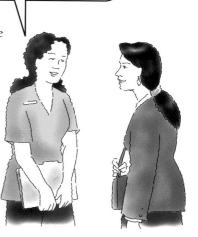

Mrs. Baxter, if you'll just take a seat, I'll see if Dr. Wright can fit you in today.

Late Patients

Patients who arrive late for their appointments cause problems in the whole day's schedule. When this happens, kindly and patiently explain to the patient that the physician will see him as soon as possible. If the patient is consistently late, explain your office's policy on lateness to him. For example, your office policy may state that patients who are more than 15 minutes late will have to be rescheduled. It might be helpful to schedule patients who you know are usually late at the end of the day. You might also remind patients that they can call if they know they are going to be late.

Physician Delays

From time to time, the physician may call to say that she will be late. If the office is not yet open, you should call patients with appointments early in the day. Let them know that they can either come in later or reschedule for another day.

If the office is already open, let patients who are already waiting know that the physician is delayed. Give patients the choice to wait or reschedule. Patients appreciate being informed of any scheduling problems.

Missed Appointments

A missed appointment is when a patient does not keep his appointment and does not let the office know ahead of time. When this happens, try to reach the patient by phone to find out why he missed his appointment and to reschedule. If you can't reach the patient this way, send a reminder card asking the patient to call the office to reschedule. Be sure to document the missed appointment in the patient's medical record. If a patient consistently misses appointments, bring the issue to the physician's attention.

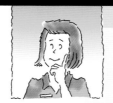

Say it Isn't So

WHAT HAPPENS WHEN THE PHYSICIAN IS DELAYED?

What are some ways to handle an office full of patients when the physician is delayed by 30 minutes or more?

The waiting room is half full and the physician has not yet arrived at the office. Finally, the physician calls to tell you she is at the hospital with a medical emergency and will be delayed by about an hour. What should you do?

Your first task is to apologize to the patients for having to wait. Then inform the patients in the waiting room that the physician has just called to say she will be delayed by about an hour. Explain that there has been a medical emergency at the hospital. Keep your voice calm and pleasant. Ask which patients would like to reschedule their appointments and who would like to stay and wait. Ask the patients who want to reschedule to come up one at a time to do so.

Cancellations

If the physician is ill, has an emergency, or is going to take time off, you may have to cancel a patient's appointment. Depending on when the situation occurs, you'll do this by phone or in writing. It's not necessary to tell patients why the physician is going to be unavailable. Simply state, "Dr. Mendez will not be available on that date," and reschedule the appointment. Be sure to note the cancellation in the patient's medical record.

If a patient needs to cancel an appointment, ask the reason and note it in the patient's medical record. Ask if the patient would like to reschedule. If a patient cancels frequently, bring this to the attention of the physician.

Referrals and Consultations

A patient may need to see another physician when his physician makes a referral or requests a consultation. A **referral** is when a patient's care is transferred to a specialist. For example, a patient with an ingrown toenail may be referred by his family doctor to a podiatrist (a physician who specializes in foot care).

A **consultation** is a request for the opinion of another physician. For example, an orthopedist may send a patient with rheumatoid arthritis to a rheumatologist for medication suggestions. The orthopedist continues to see the patient based on the rheumatologist's recommendations.

TEACHING ABOUT MEDICAL OFFICE PROCEDURES

Many patients may need to have certain tests or procedures done in the medical office. When this happens, you'll need to provide the patient with instructions about the procedure. Often, the patient will need to prepare for the procedure ahead of time. Make sure the patient understands any special instructions. Encourage the patient to ask questions.

Diagnostic Testing

Diagnostic testing such as magnetic resonance imaging (MRI), computed tomography, laboratory tests, nuclear medicine studies, or radiology procedures may need to be done at another medical facility. These appointments are usually made while the patient is still at the office. Give the patient a reminder card and referral slip with the name, address, and phone number of the other facility. If the patient's preparations for the diagnostic test are complicated, give the instructions both verbally and in writing.

Surgery

From time to time, you'll need to schedule surgical procedures for a patient that take place in a hospital or outpatient surgical facility. In some cases, you may also need to get precertification information from the patient's insurance carrier. Give a copy of the preadmission form to the patient. Make sure the patient knows to return the completed form to the hospital or facility. Also remind the patient of any diagnostic testing or laboratory work that has to be done before the surgery. Write down all appointment dates, times, and locations for the patient.

Here you go, Mrs. Adams. I've written down everything you need to do before your surgery.

Community Resources

The community offers a variety of resources to satisfy the needs of its citizens. Part of your role as medical assistant is to be aware of the community resources available to your patients. By knowing what resources are available, you can give patients the information they need to help satisfy their health needs.

TYPES OF REFERRALS

Physicians can make referrals to a variety of different people or places. A physician may refer a patient to another physician, to a community health nursing service, to a hospital emergency department, to a program for a particular health condition or disease, or to a community support group.

COMMUNITY AGENCIES

Some common community agencies include Meals on Wheels, hospice, rehabilitation services, counseling services, and the Office on Aging. Each of these agencies also has resources to which they can refer people.

Meals on Wheels

Meals on Wheels is a program that delivers one balanced meal per day to a person's home 5 days a week. This program helps meet the nutritional needs of people who have difficulty getting out of the house or who can't cook for themselves.

Hospice

Hospice Foundation of America is a national program that offers support to patients who are dying and to the patients' families and friends. Most cities have a hospice agency. Hospice care usually begins when the patient has 6 months or less to live. The hospice agency continues to provide support services to the family for one year after the patient's death. Hospice care can take place in the privacy of the patient's home or in a hospital or nursing home.

Rehabilitation Facilities

A rehabilitation facility is a community resource that specializes in services for patients who require physical or emotional rehabilitation. This type of resource also offers support to people seeking treatment for chemical dependency. The rehabilitation center usually includes a team of physicians, nurses, physical therapists, occupational therapists, and counselors.

Counseling Services

Some patients may need to see a counselor in a specific field. This counselor may be a trained mental health professional, a psychiatrist, a psychologist, a social worker, a member of the clergy, a financial counselor, a sex therapist, or an occupational therapist. As you can see, there are many different kinds of counselors. As a medical assistant, you should be aware of the circumstances in which the physician might refer a patient to one of these counselors.

Area Office on Aging

One other community resource that is available to patients is your area's Office on Aging. This agency can provide many links to services for older adults regarding transportation, hospice, home health, social groups, and other useful resources.

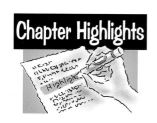

Chapter Highlights

- Patients can learn from the cognitive, affective, or psychomotor domains.
- Three different types of learners are visual (sight) learners, auditory (hearing) learners, and tactile (touch) learners; each of these types requires a different teaching approach.
- Teaching styles, educational tools, and materials should be adapted to accommodate the learning styles and needs of patients.
- Health maintenance and disease prevention strategies include understanding medical issues, providing information about community resources, using handouts, and helping patients maintain a healthy lifestyle.

- Stress has a physiological and an emotional impact on the human body. Many medical issues arise as a result of long-term stress.
- Coping methods for dealing with stress include avoiding stressors, limiting activities, talking to someone, exercising, getting proper nutrition, redirecting negative energy, and relaxing.
- Good nutrition and exercise are important for maintaining a healthy lifestyle and reducing stress.
- Medications are used to treat particular ailments and diseases. When taken properly, medications help patients maintain their health.
- Office guidelines that relate to patients include procedures for missed appointments, emergency changes and cancellations, physician delays, appointment reminders, and referrals and consultations.
- Diagnostic testing such as MRI, computed tomography, laboratory tests, nuclear medicine studies, and radiology procedures may occur in a medical office.
- Community resources that are available to patients may include Meals on Wheels, hospice agencies, rehabilitation facilities, counseling services, and offices on aging.

Active Learning

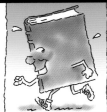

PATIENT EDUCATION BOOKLET

Work with a group to develop a patient education booklet. Choose between one of two topics:

- different community resources that may be helpful to patients
- stress and its impact on the human body

Make sure the information in the booklet is accurate and informative, but accessible to patients who may not have extensive medical knowledge. Avoid using technical terms or medical jargon. If you choose to do the booklet on community resources, be sure to include contact information for each organization along with other pertinent information. If you choose to do the stress booklet, include a section on techniques for minimizing stress. In either case, make the booklet informative and user-friendly.

CUSTOMIZED TEACHING PLAN

Work with a group to develop a teaching plan that is designed to target a specific age group or a certain type of learner (for example, auditory, visual, tactile). The teaching plan can be for a condition or treatment plan of your choosing. If you work on a teaching plan for a specific age group, be sure that the language is geared toward that group. For example, use small words and short sentences for a presentation designed for children. If you choose to work on a presentation for a specific learning type, include supplements that are designed to address the needs of that particular type of learner. In either case, remember to keep your audience in mind as you prepare the teaching plan.

Chapter 8

WRITTEN COMMUNICATIONS AND TECHNOLOGY

Chapter Checklist

- State the importance of written communication and documentation

- Explain why written communication skills are essential to the professional development of the medical assistant

- Demonstrate understanding of computer technology

- Describe the impact of computer technology on the medical office

- Discuss the use of computerized patient records

- Discuss the value of the Internet, intranet, and e-mail in the medical office

- Discuss the value of using a variety of communication equipment such as phones, fax machines, and TTY devices in the medical office

- List the components of developing an effective patient brochure that will enhance communication between the patient and the health care practice

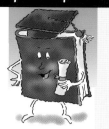

Chapter Competencies

- Explain general office policies and procedures (CAAHEP Competency 3.c.3.a.; ABHES Competency 7.a.)
- Utilize computer software to maintain office systems (CAAHEP Competency 3.c.4.c.)
- Demonstrate proper phone techniques (CAAHEP Competency 3.c.1.d.; ABHES Competency 2.e.)
- Respond to and initiate written communication (CAAHEP Competency 5.c.1.a.)
- Use correct grammar, spelling, and formatting techniques in written works (ABHES Competency 2.j.)
- Demonstrate fundamental writing skills (ABHES Competency 2.o.)

As a medical assistant, much of your communication will be in written form. Your ability to write well is an important skill. Written communications such as documents, memoranda, instructions, letters, reports, and meeting minutes must be clear, concise, and correct. You have already learned about the importance of efficient verbal communication. But efficient written communication is just as important. All your written communications should reflect positively on you, the physician, and the office.

In this chapter, you'll learn the basics of writing in the professional setting. You'll learn what information to include in medical records, how to use computers for your written communication, how to use different kinds of communication equipment, and how to create a brochure for patients.

Written Communication Is Important

As a medical assistant, you must always remember that you're a professional. All of your communications with patients—verbal and written—should therefore be professional as well. For example, a patient reminder card should not say, "Hi! Drop by and see us some time!" This tone is too casual and does not display professionalism or generate respect. Letters to patients should not have misspelled words or other mistakes. If you want patients to view you as a professional, your written communication to them must be professional.

PROFESSIONAL WRITING SKILLS

Professional writing is different from writing notes or letters to friends. The information you present in a professional letter should be easy to understand, accurate, and concise. It should not include any slang terms or colloquial phrases. For example, beginning a letter to a patient with the greeting "What's up?" or "What's new?" is unprofessional. Ending the letter with "See ya soon" or "Catch ya later" is also unprofessional.

> Professional letters should be easy to understand, accurate, and concise.

Spelling

Not everyone is a spelling bee champ. Some people are naturally good spellers. Others have to work at it. If spelling does not come naturally to you, remember that you can develop good spelling skills with time and practice.

Basic Tips

When you're unsure about the spelling of a word, look it up in a dictionary. Here are some basic tips to help you prevent spelling mistakes:

- Remember this rhyme: *i* comes before *e*, except after *c*, or when sounded like *a* as in *neighbor* and *weigh*. Exceptions are *neither, either, leisure,* and *conscience.*

Say it Isn't So

WRITING PERSONAL NOTES TO PATIENTS

What if a patient also happens to be a friend? Would it be acceptable to include a personal note on any professional communication sent from the medical office?

You may have friends, family members, or acquaintances who come to your office to see the physician. Because they are patients, it's also probable that there will be situations in which you need to send a letter, note, or other written communication to them. You should not write differently to patients who are friends. As a medical assistant, you should write just as professionally to all patients, whether you know them personally or not.

- For words ending in *ie,* drop the *e* and change the *i* to *y* before adding *ing.* Examples: *die, dying; lie, lying.*

- For words ending in *o* that are preceded by a vowel, add *s* to make them plural. Example: *studio, studios; trio, trios.* For words ending in *o* that are preceded by a consonant, add *es* to make them plural. Examples: *potato, potatoes; hero, heroes.*

- For words ending in *y* that are preceded by a vowel, add *s* to make them plural. Examples: *attorney, attorneys; day, days.* For words ending in *y* that are preceded by a consonant, change the *y* to *i* and add *es* to make them plural. Examples: *berry, berries; lady, ladies.*

- For words ending in a silent *e,* generally drop the *e* before adding a suffix beginning with a vowel. Examples: *ice, icing; judge, judging.* Exceptions are *dye, eye, shoe,* and *toe.* Do not drop the *e* when adding a suffix that begins with a consonant, unless another vowel precedes the final *e.* Examples: *pale, paleness; argue, argument.*

- For one-syllable words that end in a consonant, double the final consonant before adding a suffix beginning with a vowel. Examples: *run, running; pin, pinning.* If the final consonant is preceded by another consonant or by two vowels, do not double the consonant. Examples: *look, looked; act, acting.*

- For words ending in *c,* insert a *k* before adding a suffix beginning with *e, i,* or *y.* Examples: *picnic, picnicking; traffic, trafficker.*

Commonly Misspelled Words

There are several words in the medical field that are frequently misspelled. Some words are easily confused with words that have a similar spelling but a very different meaning. These errors can confuse communications and send the wrong message. You might want to make a list of commonly misspelled words. Put the list in a place where you can refer to it easily and quickly:

- anoxia and anorexia
- aphagia and aphasia
- bowl and bowel
- emphysema and empyema
- fundus and fungus
- lactose and lactase
- metatarsals and metacarpals

- mucus and mucous
- parental and parenteral
- postnatal and postnasal
- public and pubic
- rubella and rubeola
- serum and sebum
- uvula and vulva

Always remember to read over your documents slowly and carefully—your computer can't catch every mistake!

Spell Check

Computers make it easy to correct spelling mistakes using a spell check tool. There is even specific spell check software available for medical terminology. However, keep in mind that a spell check tool only checks for spelling errors. If you use the wrong word in a sentence, spell check will not correct it. So even if you use spell check for a document you write, make sure you read it over carefully, too.

Punctuation

Like the rules used for spelling, there are many rules about proper punctuation. You may want to make a reference list of the following punctuation symbols for yourself.

Period

A period (.) marks the end of a sentence that is a statement or a command. Examples: Get my umbrella. I'm taking a break now. Periods also follow some abbreviations such as etc., e.g., and i.e.

Question Mark

A question mark (?) marks the end of a sentence that asks a question. Examples: Where did I put my umbrella? When can I take my break?

Exclamation Point

An exclamation point (!) marks the end of a sentence that expresses great emotion. Examples: I've lost my umbrella! I forgot to take my break! Exclamation points are rarely used in professional documents.

Colon

You can use a colon (:) in different ways. You can use a colon to introduce a series of items. Example: You may use the following methods to reduce pain in your leg: (1) elevate the leg; (2) apply ice packs to the leg; and (3) take pain medication as directed by your physician.

You can use a colon following a **salutation,** or greeting, in a letter. Example:

Dear Mr. Krebs:
I am writing to inform you of the result of your recent laboratory test.

You can use a colon to separate hours and minutes. Example: Your next appointment is on July 7 at 2:30 P.M.

You can also use a colon after a heading. Example: FAMILY HISTORY: The patient reports no family history of cancer.

Semicolon

You can use a semicolon (;) to separate items that have commas within individual items on the list. Example: I visited three cities this summer: San Diego, California; Phoenix, Arizona; and Albuquerque, New Mexico.

You an also use a semicolon to connect two separate sentences. Example: I am going to get my umbrella; it's hanging on the coat rack.

Quotation Marks

Use quotation marks (" ") to set off spoken words or direct quotes. Example: When I get to the office in the morning, I usually greet my coworkers by saying, "Hi, everyone!"

Also use quotation marks to indicate the title of journal and newspaper articles. Example: The article "How to Handle Pain" in our professional journal has some good strategies for pain management.

Comma

You can use a comma (,) to separate words or phrases that are part of a series of three or more. Example: I used red, blue, green, and yellow marking pens for the demonstration.

You can also use a comma after a long introductory clause in a sentence. Example: After you fill out the paperwork with your current information, mail it back to the office.

Parentheses

Use a set of parentheses [( )] to show a part of a sentence that is not part of the main sentence but is part of the meaning of the sentence. Example: I hung my umbrella (the one I use only for work) on the coat rack.

Grammar

As you learn the rules about writing, you may become overwhelmed at how much there is to know. But do not be discouraged! The more you practice, the faster you'll memorize these rules. Soon you'll be using them automatically.

Sentence Structure

Use the following tips to write clear, well structured sentences:

- *Be concise.* Be concise and avoid long run-on sentences. For example, try to avoid writing sentences such as this one: "When I come to work in the morning I put my umbrella in the coat rack by the front entrance, then I get myself a cup of coffee and say hello to my coworkers, and then check the schedule to see which patients I am seeing that day." This sentence can be fixed like this: "When I come to work in the morning, I put my umbrella in the coat rack by the front entrance. After that, I get myself a cup of coffee and say hello to my coworkers. Finally, I check the schedule to see which patients I am seeing that day."

- *Check subjects and verbs.* Make sure the verb in a sentence agrees with the subject both in number and in person. For example, in the sentence "John carry lots of books," the subject (John) is singular—there is just one John. But the verb (carry) is plural. The subject and verb do not *agree.* This sentence should be "John carries lots of books."

- *Pay attention to tense.* The tense of a verb shows at what time the action in the sentence takes place. For example, "I went to the store" is in the past tense, and "I will go to the store" is in the future tense. The verb tenses used in a document should be consistent. For example, the following sentence has confusing verb tenses: "When you arrive at the office please give the receptionist your medical card, then took a seat and waited to be called." The sentence can be changed to read: "When you arrive at the office, please give the receptionist your medical card and then take a seat and wait to be called."

Capitalization

The first word in a sentence is always capitalized. This means that the first letter of the word is in uppercase, not lowercase. The names of proper nouns such as people, places, and holidays are also capitalized. Example: The office will be closed for Thanksgiving.

Many medical terms have unusual capitalization rules. For example, the term m-BACOD is a very different medication regimen from M-BACOD. It's critical to use the right capitalization for the circumstances. Other capitalized terms to be aware of are: pH, RhoGAM, rPA, ReoPro, and aVR.

Accuracy

Remember that information in a patient's record is permanent. Anything you write in this record must be accurate. In other words, the details must be correct. Failure to write down information accurately can result in injury or even lawsuits.

When the physician asks you to draft a letter, do not edit or rearrange the information given to you by the physician. For example, if the physician has written, "Patient was told to take Dristan Cold tablets" do not rearrange this to read, "The patient had a cold and was told to take Dristan tablets." Dristan Cold tablets are very different from regular Dristan tablets. Always ask about any information you're unfamiliar with. And be extra careful about editing any information or notes you use to compose documents.

COMPOSING DOCUMENTS

When you think of composing documents, the first thing that might come to mind is writing letters. As a medical assistant, you'll need to compose letters. Knowing how to write a letter is the basis of your ability to compose documents. However, you'll also compose many other kinds of documents such as memoranda, agendas, and meeting minutes. This section will discuss how to compose each of these documents correctly.

Letters

Writing an effective letter takes practice. There are many parts of a business letter. And just as you learned with grammar and spelling, there are certain rules that should be followed when composing a well-written, professional letter.

Components of a Business Letter

The letters you write as a medical assistant are not personal letters; they are business letters. A typical business letter has 11 components, or parts. An example of a business letter is shown on page 250. Refer to this illustration as you read the description of each component below.

1. *Letterhead.* The letterhead contains the name of the practice or physician, address, phone number, fax number, website or e-mail address of the practice, and sometimes the company logo. The letterhead may be in color and is usually centered at the top of the page.

2. *Date.* The date should include the current month, day, and year. It's typed on one line and is set two to four spaces below the letterhead. Do not use abbreviations in the date.

3. *Inside address.* The inside address is the name and address of the person to whom the letter is being sent. A zip code should also be included if possible. The inside address is usually set four spaces down from the date. Do not abbreviate city or town names, or business titles. For example, do not write CEO for Chief Executive Officer. However, abbreviating state names with the appropriate two-letter U.S. Postal Service abbreviation is preferred.

4. *Subject line.* A subject line may or may not be included in a letter. If it is, it's placed on the third line below the inside address. The subject line states the purpose of the letter. It should begin with *Re* (*Re* is an abbreviation for *regarding*). The subject should follow a colon after Re. For example, Re: blood tests.

5. *Salutation.* A salutation is the greeting of the letter. It's set two spaces down from the inside address or the subject line. The first letter of each word in the salutation should be capitalized. The salutation ends with a colon. If writing to a physician, be sure to include the person's title.

6. *Body.* The body of the letter is where the main message is. The body should be single-spaced with double-spacing between the paragraphs.

7. *Closing.* The closing is what brings the letter to an end. Some letters close with *Sincerely,* but they can also close with *Cordially yours, Respectfully, Regards,* or *Yours truly.* Only the first word in the closing is capitalized. A comma is placed after the closing.

8. *Signature and typed name.* The signature is the name of the person sending the letter. The typed name is the signature typed out. It's placed four spaces below the closing. The sender's title is typed right below the typed name. The signature goes directly above the typed name. Sometimes, you may be instructed to sign a letter for the physician. In this case, you would sign the physician's name followed by a slash mark and your name. For example, Susan James, M.D./Raymond Smith, RMA.

9. *Identification line.* The identification line may or may not be included in a business letter. It shows who dictated the letter and who wrote it. It's always abbreviated. The initials of the person who dictated the letter are capitalized, followed by the lowercase initials of the writer.

10. *Enclosure.* An enclosure is something that is included with the letter. It could be another document, a bro-

chure, or some other piece of information. If there is an enclosure, it's indicated by the abbreviation *Enc.* placed two spaces down from the identification line. If there is more than one enclosure, the number of enclosures is shown in parentheses.

11. *Copy.* The abbreviation *c* indicates that a duplicate, or copy, of the letter has been sent. Copies of letters are often sent to managers, supervisors, or the physician who dictated the letter. The copy abbreviation is placed two spaces below the enclosure line.

Format

There are three basic types of formats used for letters. They are: full block, block, and semiblock. The type of format you use is determined by office policy or by the physician's preference.

- In **block format,** all lines are flush left. This means that all lines are even with the left margin and are not indented. This is the most common and the most formal type of format. The sample business letter on page 250 is written in block format.

- In **modified block format,** the date, subject line, closing, and signature are aligned at the center or to the right of center. All other lines are flush left.

- In **modified semiblock format,** the first sentence of each paragraph is indented five spaces, or tabbed once. The date, subject line, closing, and signature are aligned at the center or to the right of center.

Composition Goals

When you compose a letter, you should have three goals:

- to write clearly

- to write concisely

- to write accurately

Composing a letter with these three goals in mind will help you write a well-written letter that is easy for the reader to understand.

A clear message is exact and precise. When the message is clear, the reader has no doubt about what is being said. For example, the statement "Contact the office" is not clear or precise. "Contact the office by Wednesday, July 20" is more precise and clearly states the message.

A concise message is short and to the point. Unnecessary words make a message long and confusing. For example, "Please enclose a personal or business check in the amount of exactly $50" is not concise. "Please enclose a $50 check" is clear and concise.

Benjamin Matthews, M.D.
999 Oak Road, Suite 313
Middletown, Connecticut 06457
860-344-6000

February 2, 2009

Dr. Adam Meza
Medical Director
Family Practice Associates
134 N. Tater Drive
West Hartford, Connecticut 06157

Re: Ms. Beatrice Suess

Dear Dr. Meza:

Thank you for asking me to evaluate Ms. Suess. I agree with your diagnosis of rheumatoid arthritis. Her prodromal symptoms include vague articular pain and stiffness, weight loss and general malaise. Ms. Suess states that the joint discomfort is most prominent in the mornings, gradually improving throughout the day.

My physical examination shows a 40-year-old female patient in good health. Heart sounds normal, no murmurs or gallops noted. Lung sounds clear. Enlarged lymph nodes were noted. Abdomen soft, bowel sounds present, and the spleen was not enlarged. Extremities showed subcutaneous nodules and flexion contractures on both hands.

Laboratory findings were indicative of rheumatoid arthritis. See attached laboratory data. I do not feel x-rays are warranted at this time.

My recommendations are to continue Ms. Suess on salicylate therapy, rest and physical therapy. I suggest that you have Ms. Suess attend physical therapy at the American Rehabilitation Center on Main Street.

Thank you for this interesting consultation.

Yours truly,

Benjamin Matthews, MD
Benjamin Matthews, MD   ⑧

BM/es   ⑨

Enc. (2)   ⑩

cc: Dr. Samuel Adams   ⑪

A typical business letter has 11 components.

An accurate message gives the correct date, time, location, address, or other information. "Your appointment is at 12:15 on Thursday, July 10" is not accurate if the appointment is really at 12:30 and July 10 is a Wednesday, not a Thursday.

Editing and Proofreading

Even after your letter is written, you still have some work to do. Editing a document is a key step in writing successfully. Look over the letter for errors in grammar, spelling, and content. There are two steps to proper editing—proofreading and making corrections. You may ask a coworker to help you proofread a document to make sure it's accurate and easy to understand. A proofreader gives you feedback about a document. Here are items a proofreader should look for:

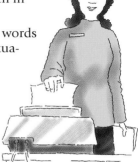

After you have made corrections, print out a final copy of your letter.

- *Accuracy.* All information should be correct and precise.
- *Clarity and conciseness.* Information should be written in clear, concise sentences.
- *Spelling, grammar, punctuation, and capitalization.* All words should be spelled correctly. Correct grammar, punctuation, and capitalization rules should be followed.
- *Logical flow.* The information in the letter should be well organized and flow in a logical way.

After the proofreader edits your letter, make corrections to your document and print a final copy. You might want to read over the final copy one last time to make sure you do not miss any errors or forget to make any corrections.

Mailing the Letter

After the final copy of the letter has been printed, all that remains is to mail it out. The size of a standard business envelope is 4 1/8 by 9 1/2 inches. Once the letter is ready to go, there are several options for mailing. These include:

- *Express Mail.* This is the fastest delivery option, which ensures delivery by the next day. Rates vary by weight and destination, and the mail is automatically insured for $500 with additional insurance available.
- *Priority Mail.* This option offers two- or three-day delivery to most destinations for letters and packages weighing up to 70 pounds. Rates vary based on the weight of the package, and insurance is available.
- *First-Class Mail.* This option is generally used for sending standard mail items such as letters and post cards. Anything that weighs more than 13 ounces, however, is considered Priority Mail.

- *Standard Mail.* This is the slowest delivery option, typically used by companies to mail books, catalogs, or other packages weighing less than 16 ounces that do not require speedy delivery. However, Standard Mail can't be used to send letters or billing statements.

You also have the option of sending First-Class and Priority Mail items as Certified Mail, which provides a mailing receipt and a record of the mailing at the local post office. Certified mail is useful for sending out important documents and can be used to confirm that the recipient actually received them.

Keep in mind that postal rates, fees, and services are subject to change. Visit www.usps.com for additional information and updates.

Memoranda

A **memorandum** is a note or letter used for communication within the office or between departments. It's also called a memo. Memoranda are not formal and are usually used for short announcements. The parts of a memorandum are described in the list below.

- *Heading.* The word "Memorandum" is typed across the top of the page as a heading. It's sometimes abbreviated as "Memo." This lets the reader know that the document is a memorandum and not a letter.
- *Date.* The rules for writing the date on a memorandum are the same as those for a letter.
- *To.* After the word *To* and a colon, list all the names of those receiving the memorandum. These names should be in either alphabetical or hierarchic order. If you send the memorandum to an entire group or department, you can address the memorandum to the name of that group or department. For example, To: Marketing Department.
- *From.* After the word *From* and a colon, list the name and title of the person sending the memorandum.
- *Subject.* The subject is a brief statement describing the purpose of the memorandum. For example, Subject: Today's Staff Meeting.
- *Body.* The body is where you write the actual message of the memorandum.
- *Copy.* The copy indicates who is receiving copies of the memorandum. Use the *c* just as you learned in the section on writing letters.

Franklin Dermatology Center
123 Main Street
Rockfall, Kansas
913-755-2600

Memorandum
To: All Medical Assistants
From: Patty Stricker, Office Manager
Date: 12/03/09
Re: Holiday time

Please notify me by December 10 of any requests you have for taking time off during Christmas or New Year's. Remember that holiday requests will be based on seniority. The office will be closed at noon on December 24. The office will be closed on the 25th and reopen on the 26th. The office will also close on December 31st at noon. The office will be closed on January 1, reopening on the 2nd.

If you have any questions, please e-mail me.

A memorandum is less formal than a business letter
and is generally used for brief announcements.

Agendas

An **agenda** is a brief outline of the topics to be discussed at a meeting. Having an agenda makes it easier for people at a meeting to know what to expect. It helps make the meeting more organized and efficient. Handing out an agenda on the day before a meeting helps participants prepare for the meeting. An agenda should have the following parts:

- call to order
- review and acceptance of the minutes from [insert date of last meeting]
- old business
- new business
- adjournment

Quality Improvement Committee
February 15, 2009
Agenda

I. Call to order
II. Review and acceptance of the minutes from January 10, 2009
III. Old business
   A. Copy machine updates
   B. Insurance updates for overdue accounts
IV. New business
   A. New contract for laboratory supplies
   B. Scheduling guidelines for summer vacations
V. Adjournment

Agendas usually begin with a call to order, followed by a review of previous meeting minutes, old business updates, then new business. Adjournment is the last item on the agenda.

Meeting Minutes

Everything that takes place at a meeting is recorded in the meeting minutes. You should always type up meeting minutes as soon as possible after a meeting. Include the following information in the meeting minutes:

- list of members at the meeting
- list of members who were absent
- date and time the meeting was called to order

- statement about whether or not the previous minutes were accepted
- brief description of discussions
- action items and responsible party
- list of any reports that were submitted
- date and time of the next meeting
- adjournment time
- signature of the person who prepared the minutes and the chairperson's signature

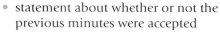

An agenda helps keep a meeting organized.

THE MEDICAL RECORD

A medical record contains confidential clinical information about the patient's health and treatment. It also includes information about insurance and billing. Today, many offices use an electronic system for maintaining patient records. If your office has not yet switched to an electronic medical records system, you'll use a different way of organizing and keeping records.

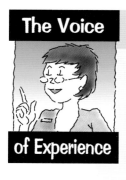

The Voice of Experience

THE MEDICAL RECORD

Q: *What is the best way to file and maintain medical records?*

A: Every medical office has its own system for maintaining records. Regardless of the system, there are certain general guidelines to follow regarding medical records.

- Make sure office personnel can get to the records easily.
- Keep the records neat and orderly.
- Make sure the information in all records is complete.
- Make sure the records are easy to read.
- Check that all information in medical records is accurate.
- Write medical information concisely and clearly.

Contents

A medical record contains a patient's general information, including her name, address, phone number, date of birth, Social Security number, credit history, and emergency contacts. But the record also contains confidential clinical information about the patient's health and treatment. Billing and insurance information is included in the medical record, too.

General Information

As you can probably imagine, there is a lot of information in a patient's medical record. How is so much information organized in one chart? To organize patient information, you can use metal fasteners to keep general information on one side of the chart and medical information on the other side.

Clinical Section

The medical, or clinical, information in a patient's record usually contains the following:

- *Chief complaint.* This is the original reason or set of symptoms that led the patient to see the physician. The chief complaint is usually recorded in quotation marks with the patient's own words. For example, the patient might say, "The right side of my head was hurting."

- *Present illness.* This is information about the onset and characteristics of the patient's illness. For example, the headache, which is dull and throbbing, started two days ago, and ordinary Tylenol was taken with no relief.

- *Family and personal history.* This is a review of any illnesses in the patient's family members. The patient's previous illnesses and surgeries are listed here.

- *Systems review.* This is a review of the major body systems to see if any other problems might exist. For example, a change in a mole might indicate a problem with the integumentary system.

- *Progress notes.* This is documentation of each patient encounter, including information obtained in phone calls and refills of prescriptions.

- *Radiographic reports.* This is information about any x-rays or other radiographic procedures that the patient has had done.

- *Lab results.* This includes a copy of any laboratory work that the patient has had done.

- *Consultation reports.* This is information from other physicians regarding the patient's health and treatment.

- *Diagnosis or medical impression.* This information contains the physician's opinion about the patient's problems.
- *Physician, nurse, and/or medical assistant signature.* Any medical professional who consults with, interviews, or treats the patient should include his complete signature in this section.
- *Advance directives and power of attorney.* This is information about any instructions from the patient regarding end-of-life decisions, power of attorney, or particular persons who can give consent for treatment of the patient.
- *HIPAA.* This is the Health Insurance Portability and Accountability Act. This law helps protect and regulate health insurance coverage. It also helps protect the patient's privacy.
- *Correspondence.* The patient's medical record also contains copies of any letters or memoranda regarding the patient's health care. The person who wrote the letters and memoranda should sign them.

Abbreviations and Symbols

As a medical assistant, you should be familiar with and know how to use abbreviations in a patient's medical record. You'll find that using abbreviations and symbols saves a lot of time and space.

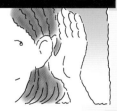

Listen to This

ABBREVIATIONS AND SYMBOLS

Here is a list of some common abbreviations to use when recording patient information. Memorize as many of these as you can. You'll use some of these abbreviations more often than others.

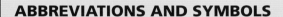

Commonly Used Medical Abbreviations

Abbreviation	Meaning	Abbreviation	Meaning
ac	before meals	AM, a.m., A.M.	morning
ad lib	as desired	amp	ampule
ADL	activities of daily living	amt	amount
		aq	aqueous

Abbreviation	Meaning	Abbreviation	Meaning
bid	twice a day	NS	normal saline
BM	bowel movement	OD	right eye
		OS	left eye
BRP	bathroom privileges	OU	both eyes
		os	mouth
c̄	with	oz	ounce
cap	capsule	p	after
DC, disc, d/c	discontinue	pc	after meals
disp	dispense	PM, p.m., P.M.	afternoon or evening
DW	distilled water		
EDC	estimated date of confinement (date baby is due)	po, PO	by mouth
		prn, PRN	whenever necessary
et	and	pt	pint or patient
ext	extract	q	every
FGW	full glass of water	qh	every hour
		q2h	every 2 hours
FU	follow up	q3h	every 3 hours
g, gm	gram	qid	four times a day
gr	grain	qt	quart
gt(t)	drop(s)	R	right, rectal
h, hr	hour	RTW	return to work
hs, HS	hour of sleep	Rx	take, prescribe
ID	intradermal	s̄	without
IM	intramuscular	SC, subcu, subq, S/Q, SQ	subcutaneously
IV	intravenous	Sig	label
kg	kilogram	SL	sublingual
L, l	liter	sol	solution
lb	pound	SOS	once if necessary
LMP	last menstrual period	ss	one-half
		stat, STAT	immediately
mcg, μg	microgram	supp	suppository
mEq	milliequivalent	syr	syrup
ml, mL	milliliter	tab	tablet
n	normal	T, tb, tbs, tbsp	tablespoon
NaCl	sodium chloride	t, tsp	teaspoon
NH	nursing home	tid	three times a day
NKA	no known allergies	WNL	within normal limits
Noc	night		
NPO	nothing by mouth		

Formats

There are different formats for recording and documenting patient information. The three most common formats used in medical offices are:

- **SOAP,** which includes *subjective, objective, assessment*, and *planning* notes
- **problem-oriented medical record (POMR),** which lists each problem of the patient, usually at the beginning of the folder, and references each problem with a number throughout the folder
- **narrative,** which is simply a paragraph indicating the contact with the patient, what was done for the patient, and the outcome of any action

How Computer Technology Helps

Computers have many purposes in the medical office. They can make certain tasks easier. Most medical offices use computers and computer programs for everyday office procedures, such as scheduling, billing, and insurance filing. In the medical office, you may also use computers for clinical procedures such as reading laboratory and radiology reports, creating and updating patient records, and writing medication orders.

COMPUTER HARDWARE, PERIPHERALS, AND SOFTWARE

A computer system is divided into parts—the hardware, the peripherals, and the software. Learning about these parts will help you understand the computer system as a whole.

Hardware

The equipment and machinery that make up the computer are called the computer's **hardware.** These are things that are part of the basic computer system. Hardware includes the CPU (central processing unit), keyboard, monitor, and hard drive.

Peripherals

The **peripherals** of the computer system are things that are connected to or plugged into the basic computer system from the outside. Some examples of peripherals include an external **modem** for connecting to the Internet, a mouse, a scanner, a printer, and battery backup.

Software

Software is a program or application that allows the computer system to do certain things. One software program might allow you to create patient charts. Another might help you manage patient prescriptions. As you might guess, there are many medical software programs available. Part of your job as a medical assistant is to become as familiar as possible with the software programs your medical office uses.

> Let's see, Mrs. Paxton, it looks like you have been taking this medication since last August.

COMPUTERIZED MEDICAL RECORDS

Using a computer system to create and store medical records can save time and space. Today's touch-screen technology makes it even easier to store patient information. Of course, there are both advantages and disadvantages to using computerized medical records.

Advantages

Here are some of the advantages to using a computer system to create and store patient records:

- *Saves space and paper.* Computerized records do not use paper. They also do not require the storage space that paper records do.
- *Easy to read.* Because the information in computerized records is in typeface, it's easier to read than handwriting.
- *Accessible.* Physicians and other medical personnel can easily search computerized records to gain quick access to a patient's record.
- *Easy to update.* Changes to a patient's computerized record are quick and easy to make.

Disadvantages

Here are a few disadvantages to using computerized medical records:

- *Training time.* All office personnel must be trained to use the software program. Such training takes time.
- *Security.* Patient records are easy to access when they are stored on a computer. Therefore, every office must have

policies to preserve the privacy and confidentiality of their patients' medical records.

- *Equipment failure.* An equipment breakdown or power outage can cause a computer to stop working. When a computer is not working, computerized patient records are not accessible.

INTERNET

The computer system in a medical office probably lets you access information on the World Wide Web. The network that enables you to do this is called the **Internet.**

Connection

To access the World Wide Web, your computer system must connect to the Internet. There are three ways of doing this. One is by using a phone line and an Internet service provider (ISP). A second way is through your cable television company. This kind of connection is faster than using a regular phone line. A third way of connecting to the Internet is a digital subscriber line (DSL). This is the fastest connection, but is not available everywhere. It's also the most expensive type of Internet connection.

Your web browser is a software program that lets your computer communicate with the Internet. Examples of web browsers are Internet Explorer and Mozilla Firefox.

Security

It's important that you never send any patient information over the Internet to a site that is not secure. Sites with a secure sockets layer (SSL) are secure. They scramble information that leaves your computer and unscramble it when it arrives at its destination. This keeps the information secure.

Always look for the lock icon on your computer's status bar. This indicates that the site you're looking at is secure.

Viruses

A **computer virus** is a program that can invade your computer and destroy files. A virus can do a lot of damage in a short period of time, so it's important to have effective and up-to-date virus protection software on your computer system.

Protection Software

Most computers come equipped with virus protection software. This software must be updated frequently to get the most recent and effective version.

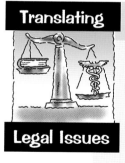

E-MAIL CONFIDENTIALITY

E-mail is a quick and convenient way to communicate with others in your office. But there is one important fact to keep in mind when using e-mail. The messages you send and receive can't be guaranteed to be private and confidential. To help keep your e-mail messages as confidential and private as possible, follow these tips:

- Send only work-related e-mail messages. Do not send personal messages using your work e-mail address.

- Read about your e-mail program's encryption feature and activate it. Encryption is a process that scrambles messages so that they can't be read until they reach the recipient.

- Use the out-of-office-assistant feature to alert senders when you're out of the office or on vacation. This lets senders know that you will not be reading their messages immediately.

Protection Tips

No virus protection program is perfect. Here are a few tips that will help you keep your computer system safe:

- Do not open any attachments from unknown or suspicious sites.

- Update your virus protection software regularly. Use the update option in your virus protection program daily.

- Make sure your virus protection program protects against computer worms. These can also do great damage to your system and any information stored in it.

> Update your computer's virus protection software daily.

INTRANET

An **intranet** is a private network of computers that share data, such as in a medical office. It's also called an internal web. An intranet can be especially handy in an office with many physicians.

Access

Your office's intranet access is limited to the people who work there. In other words, only the people who work within the office can use it. However, you may be able to access your office's intranet from a home computer.

Benefits

The advantage of your office's intranet is that it makes it easier to communicate with everyone you work with. As a result, communication between those who work at your office is stronger and more effective. Good communication can help many tasks get done faster.

Common Examples of Intranet Data

There are many kinds of data that can be sent and received over the office intranet. They include:

- information about policies and procedures
- marketing
- meeting minutes
- staff schedules
- commonly used forms
- internal newsletters
- internal job postings
- phone lists
- video conference supports
- links to important medical sites

E-MAIL

Electronic mail, or **e-mail,** is any mail sent through a computer network. E-mail messages are sent to and from computers every day. This amounts to trillions of e-mails per year! There are many benefits to using e-mail, including:

- *Better patient care.* Using e-mail to communicate with your coworkers makes it easier to get information about a patient's health care.
- *Teamwork.* Using e-mail makes it easier for those at your office to work together as a team.
- *No more phone tag.* E-mail eliminates the need to keep calling people back if they are not available to pick up the phone the first time you call.
- *Written documentation.* E-mail provides written documentation of information.

Composing Messages

When composing a professional e-mail, follow the guidelines for writing business letters. In addition, keep the following in mind:

- Check your spelling, grammar, and punctuation before sending any e-mail messages.

- Keep your e-mail messages short and concise.
- If an e-mail message is important, flag it to alert the person you're sending it to. However, never send e-mail about a patient who is in an emergency situation. Always call or page a physician in an emergency situation.
- Use appropriate fonts and font sizes in your e-mail.
- Use generic or plain stationery for all e-mails.
- Always fill in the subject line of e-mail messages.
- Limit each e-mail message to one topic.
- Do not indent the paragraphs of e-mail messages.
- If you like, add a permanent signature to your outgoing e-mail messages.
- Add the recipient's e-mail address last to avoid sending any unfinished e-mails by mistake.

> To: Steve Warner <s_warner@email.com>
> From: Carla Sanchez <Carla.Sanchez@medicalgroup.com>
> Date: 26 Feb 2009
> Subject: Records Transfer Request
>
> Dear Mr. Warner,
>
> Your medical records will be transfered to Dr. Wen's office this afternoon, per your request. Please note that there is no fee for transferring your records to another physician.
>
> Please don't hesitate to contact Family Medical Group if you need anything else. I can be reached by phone at (555) 123-1000 or by email at Carla.Sanchez@medicalgroup.com.
>
> Best regards,
>
> Carla Sanchez, CMA
>
> Family Medical Group
> 100 Medical Parkway, Suite 101
> Anytown, USA 12345
> Phone: (555) 123-1000
> Fax: (555) 123-4567
> E-mail Carla.Sanchez@medicalgroup.com
>
> *The information contained in this e-mail is confidential and intended for the sole use of the individual named above. If you are not the intended recipient, please delete this e-mail immediately.*

Here is an example of a professional e-mail.

Address Books

E-mail software has a feature that allows you to create an **address book,** or a collection of e-mail addresses. You can also add other information such as phone numbers, street addresses, and fax numbers to the address book. Make sure you keep your address book up to date. It's also helpful to keep business addresses in a separate folder from personal addresses.

Attachments

An **attachment** is a file that is sent along with an e-mail message. The file could be a document, photograph, x-ray, or chart. A single e-mail may include several attachments. Here are some guidelines to keep in mind when using attachments:

- After opening an attachment, store it immediately in an appropriate place on your computer. If needed, print out the attachment.
- To send an attachment, first write your e-mail message and then select the option for adding attachments. Find the file or document you wish to attach and click on it. It's always

a good idea to click on the attachment after you have added it to make sure it's the correct file.

Communication Equipment

Physicians use many expensive technical machines and instruments to diagnose and treat patients. You have learned about some of these. But of all the equipment in your medical office, the most important are the ones you use to communicate with others. Most medical offices have phones, fax machines, and TTYs. These machines make it easier for you and your coworkers to communicate with other medical offices, physicians, and patients.

PHONE

The phone makes it possible to schedule appointments, refill prescriptions, get test results, inquire about a patient, and report an emergency. By simply picking up the phone receiver and pushing numbers, you can quickly contact patients, coworkers, physicians, hospitals, and pharmacies. The phone links the physician's office to the patient and to the healthcare community.

It's important that others are able to understand you when you call them on the phone. Like any other piece of equipment, there are some guidelines and tips to follow when using the phone.

Yes, Mr. Ortiz, I would be happy to reschedule your appointment for you.

Speak Clearly

Speak clearly and distinctly when talking on the phone. Enunciate your words. Make sure you're speaking directly into the mouthpiece. Also make sure you're not speaking too quickly or too softly.

Pronunciation and Language

It's important to pronounce words correctly so that others understand what you're saying. Medical words and terms are new to most patients, so make sure you use them sparingly or explain what they mean when you do use them. For example, instead of asking a patient, "Are you dyspneic today?" ask "Are you having trouble breathing today?"

Smile

It may sound like a little thing, but putting a smile in your voice makes any phone conversation more effective. When you speak to others on a phone, avoid using a bored, monotonous tone.

Listen

Do not forget to listen to the person on the other end of the phone. Let the other person speak without being interrupted. If you didn't quite understand what the person said, ask him to repeat it. Offer feedback to let the speaker know you understand what he is telling you.

Be Courteous

Always speak politely and courteously with all patients and medical personnel. Avoid casual language like "Hey, Bob, how's it going today?" Instead, say "Good morning, Mr. Brown. How are you feeling today?"

FAX MACHINE

A **facsimile (fax) machine** allows your medical office to send or receive printed material over a phone line. You can send medical records, orders, prescriptions, or test results using a fax machine. Here are a few tips to help you maintain patients' confidentiality while using a fax machine:

- Before sending particularly sensitive information, contact the recipient of the fax so that he may retrieve the fax himself.
- Always use a cover sheet with a confidentiality statement.
- Make sure you never leave information you have faxed in the fax machine tray.

TTY

TTY stands for teletypewriter. It may also be called TDD, or telecommunication device for the deaf. A TTY is a device that helps people who have trouble hearing or speaking use the phone to communicate. With a TTY, people can type messages back and forth instead of talking and listening. A TTY device must be in use at both ends of a conversation to communicate this way.

Using a TTY device is easy. Post these simple steps near your office's TTY as a reminder for anybody who may need to use the TTY when using the phone.

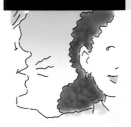

Send and Receive

PUTTING PATIENTS ON HOLD

Suppose that you receive a call from a patient who would like to reschedule an appointment. While you're speaking to the caller, another call comes in. What do you do? What is the best way to put a patient on hold? Here is an example of an ineffective and effective way to put a patient on hold.

Ineffective:

- "Good morning, Mr. Caballa. What can I do for you?"
- Mr. Caballa replies, "I need to reschedule my Wednesday appointment."
- Your phone signals you that another call is coming through. "Mr. Caballa, I have another call coming through, I'll be right back."
- Five minutes later, you're able to get back to Mr. Caballa, who is no longer on the line.

It's important that you never leave a caller on hold for more than 3 minutes. Before doing so, always ask, "Do you mind if I put you on hold?" If you must keep a caller on hold for longer than 3 minutes, ask if he would like to call back later.

Effective:

- "Good morning, Mr. Caballa. What can I do for you?"
- Mr. Caballa replies, "I need to reschedule my Wednesday appointment."
- Your phone signals you that another call is coming through. "I'm sorry, Mr. Caballa, I have another call coming through. Would you mind holding for just a minute?" You wait for Mr. Caballa to respond.
- "No, I can't really hold right now," Mr. Caballa tells you.
- "No problem, Mr. Caballa. Let me transfer you to another receptionist. She can reschedule your appointment for you."

Another option in this situation would have been to ask Mr. Caballa to call back later. Or you can offer to call him back as soon as you're free. If you feel like you're juggling phone calls and other tasks, keep as calm as possible. Use your best judgment in putting callers on hold and asking patients to wait before checking them in. Remember also that all information shared between you and a patient over the phone is confidential.

1. Set the phone handset onto the TTY's special acoustic cups.

2. Use the keyboard on the TTY to type the message you want to send.

3. Your message will be sent as you type it.

4. The other person's response to your message will appear on the TTY's text display.

If you do not have a TTY, you can still call a patient who is deaf or can't speak on the phone by using a telecommunications relay service (TRS). With this service, an operator uses a TTY device to type your message to the patient you're calling. The patient reads your message on her TTY and responds to the TRS operator. Then the operator reads the patient's response aloud to you. There are toll-free TRS services available 24 hours a day.

Patient Brochures

As a medical assistant, you may contribute to the development of a patient brochure for your medical office. This brochure contains information about what the patient can expect from the physician. It also contains information about what is expected of the patient. The patient brochure helps strengthen the communication between the patient and your medical office.

The patient brochure contains a lot of information, so it's important that it's organized and clearly presented. The following sections describe the information usually included in a patient brochure. You may include additional information, depending on your medical office and the amount of space available in the brochure.

PRACTICE NAME

The most important pieces of information in a patient brochure are the name of the medical practice, address, website, e-mail address, and phone number. The practice name should be on the front of the brochure and should be easy to see and read. You may also want to put this information on the back of the brochure. There may be places throughout the brochure where you'll want to place the phone number.

LIST OF PHYSICIANS

Below the name of the medical practice should be the names of the physicians in the office. Having a small photo of each physician is also a good idea.

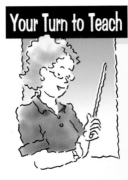

Your Turn to Teach

PATIENT BROCHURES

Your patient brochure should be colorful and easy to read. It should contain answers to questions a patient might have about your medical office. Make sure your brochures are placed in the office where patients can easily find them.

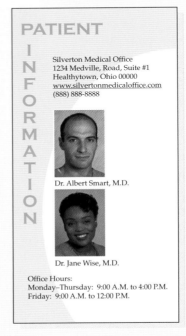

A patient brochure includes basic information about the medical practice.

OFFICE HOURS

Place the office hours where they are easy to see and understand. If the office closes for lunch, you might want to have this information printed in large letters.

DIRECTIONS

Including a small map to show patients where your medical office is located is always helpful. You might also add the office phone number near the map in case patients need further directions.

SCHEDULING AND CANCELING APPOINTMENTS

Clearly and concisely explain the procedure for scheduling and canceling an appointment. Provide the phone number again in this section so that patients do not have to look for it. If there is a separate phone number for canceling appointments, provide it here. Make sure to include how far in advance a patient should cancel an appointment to avoid being billed.

MEDICATION REFILLS

Every office has its own policy for refilling medications. Explain as concisely as possible how a patient should get his medication refilled. For some offices, the local pharmacy will call the physician for the patient. If space allows, the brochure could include a list of local pharmacy names, addresses, and phone numbers.

EMERGENCY SITUATIONS

All patients need to know what to do if they have a medical emergency and the office is closed. Usually, the regular phone number for the office will ring directly to an answering service when the office is closed. Explain in this section that during non-business hours, non–life-threatening emergencies will be handled by the physician on call. You may want to include a note here to direct patients to call 911 or go to the nearest emergency room for any serious or life-threatening emergencies.

PARKING

Most patients will drive a car to your medical office. One way to let patients know where to park is to show a picture of the medical office and available parking areas. Or the brochure might simply describe where patients can park.

It might also be helpful to include information about the nearest bus stop, taxi companies, or mass transit services.

IMPORTANT OFFICE PROCEDURES

In this section, you can explain important office procedures such as:

- how insurance is billed
- what methods of payment are accepted
- when co-payments are paid
- what to expect during an appointment
- any other diagnostic services provided by the office

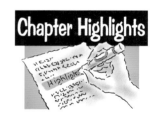

- Written communications and documentation are important ways for medical offices to interact with patients and manage office procedures.
- Good writing skills are essential for medical assistants to communicate effectively. Medical assistants must know how to write clearly, concisely, and accurately.
- Computer systems include hardware, peripherals, and software.
- Computer technology increases the efficiency of the medical office.
- Many medical offices use computerized patient records. Computerized patient records are an easy and efficient way of collecting and storing patient information.
- The Internet, intranet, and e-mail strengthen communications between those who work inside and outside the medical office.
- Using a variety of communication equipment, such as phones, fax machines, and TTY devices, makes communicating with all patients easier and more effective.
- An effective patient brochure includes the practice name; list of physicians in the practice; office hours; directions to the office; parking information; and policies on scheduling, canceling appointments, medication refills, and office procedures.

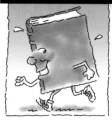

LETTER WRITING

Suppose the medical office you work in is changing its hours. The office will no longer be open on Mondays. However, it will stay open later (until 8:00 P.M.) on Wednesdays and Thursdays. Compose a business letter from your physician's practice regarding this change. In the letter, be sure to review the office hours for each day of the week. Follow the business letter format and write clearly, accurately, and professionally.

COMPUTER VIRUS PROTECTION

Use the Internet to research the most current information on computer viruses. Review how to update virus protection software on a computer.

Chapter 9

USING PROFESSIONAL COMMUNICATION SKILLS IN THE WORKPLACE

Chapter Checklist

- Use therapeutic communication skills to communicate effectively with all members of the health care team

- Demonstrate an understanding of workplace dynamics and office procedures

- List the sources of a conflict

- List the stages of a conflict

- List and describe conflict management techniques

- Identify and describe varying supervisory styles

- Develop a resume

- Describe interview strategy techniques

- State the importance of developing and employing therapeutic communication skills and techniques that enable medical assistants to grow personally and professionally

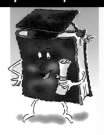

Chapter Competencies

- Recognize and respond to verbal and nonverbal communication (CAAHEP Competency 3.c.1.b. and 3.c.1.c.; ABHES Competency 2.i. and 2.l.)
- Interview effectively (ABHES Competency 2.f.)
- Be a "team player" (ABHES Competency 1.c.)
- Be courteous and diplomatic (ABHES Competency 1.h.)
- Be attentive, listen, and learn (ABHES Competency 2.a.)
- Be impartial and show empathy when dealing with patients (ABHES Competency 2.b.)
- Demonstrate fundamental writing skills (ABHES Competency 2.o.)

As a medical assistant, you'll perform many different tasks throughout the day. In fact, one of your biggest challenges is being prepared for the many situations that could occur at any time. But there is one thing you'll have to do every day with every person you work with: communicate. You've already learned about the importance of communicating effectively with patients. But what about the people you work with? Your ability to communicate with others on your health care team is also critical to your success as a medical assistant.

In this chapter, you'll learn how to communicate effectively with other members of the health care team. This will include learning how to prepare for interviews as well as using appropriate interviewing skills. You'll also learn how to approach, deal with, and resolve the many different kinds of conflicts that may arise in the workplace.

Communicating with Your Health Care Team

The office where you work includes many people. Your health care team is the most valuable part of your medical office. The people who make up your team are more important than technical knowledge, physical facilities, sophisticated equipment, or physical location. But in order for the health care team to be effective, each team member must be able to communicate effectively. Being able to communicate effectively with one another helps the entire health care team provide the best possible care for patients.

MEMBERS OF THE HEALTH CARE TEAM

Your health care team is everybody who works in your medical office. The physician, nurses, medical office manager, health care specialists, and, of course, the medical assistants, are all members of this team.

COMMUNICATION SKILLS FOR THE HEALTH CARE TEAM

The way you communicate with your coworkers should always be professional and courteous. It should be based on honesty and integrity. Communication with coworkers is not always easy. The way you communicate with team members should reflect respect for one another's knowledge and skill level. It should also adhere to your professional organization's code of ethics. Information about patients shared between coworkers should always be kept confidential.

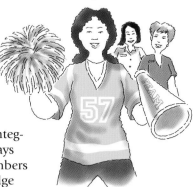

Go, team! By being a supportive member of the health care team, you can help keep the office running smoothly.

INTERDISCIPLINARY COMMUNICATIONS

You'll find that people from two or more medical specialties often work together to meet a specific goal. For example, the lab technician consults with the nurse or physician. The physician consults with the specialist to whom he referred the patient. These types of interactions are called **interdisciplinary communication**. This kind of communication builds a stronger health care team and improves the patients' care environment.

When team members communicate with one another effectively and consistently, they help create an atmosphere of collaboration. They draw on the knowledge and skills of each team member. Why is this so important? It's the unique viewpoint of each team member that makes any treatment plan more effective.

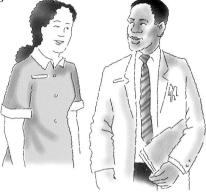

I thought you should know, Doctor, that Mr. Rivera is very concerned about his diagnosis.

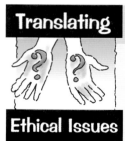

IMPAIRED COWORKERS

The National Association of Social Workers website states, "An estimated 20 percent of workers suffer from some type of impairment, which may include substance abuse, psychological stresses due to aging, physical illness, financial hardship, extreme working conditions, marital and family difficulties, or chronic psychological disorders." These impairments may create ethical situations for health care practitioners.

For example, suppose you're the office manager for a well respected family physician in a small town. He is 70 years old and is starting to show signs of senility. He is forgetful and has even been disoriented and confused a few times. No one seems to have noticed. You respect the physician, but you're concerned that his condition may be placing patients' health and safety at risk. How should you handle this ethical dilemma?

Any time a physician or coworker's impairment has the potential to affect the quality of care being provided to patients, it's your ethical responsibility to report your concerns to the appropriate authority. In this particular situation, you should report the physician's condition to the administration of the hospital where he has privileges or to the state board of medicine. The physician's family may be involved in the situation as well.

Workplace Dynamics and Office Procedures

The way you and your coworkers interact affects the success of the medical office. As you know, working as a supportive team is the goal of each employee. Understanding and following the procedures and policies of your office keep things running smoothly and efficiently.

ORGANIZATIONAL STRUCTURE

Every medical office has its own **organizational structure**. The chart on the next page illustrates where each employee fits into the structure of the medical office. The chart also represents the **chain of command** within the office. Employees should follow the chain of command to resolve any personnel issues that may arise between members of the health care team.

To perform the best job you can, you need to know what your job description entails. A job description is a written document that lists and describes the duties and expectations of a particular position. Your office manager should have a copy of the job description for every position in your medical office. Feel free to ask for a copy of your job description.

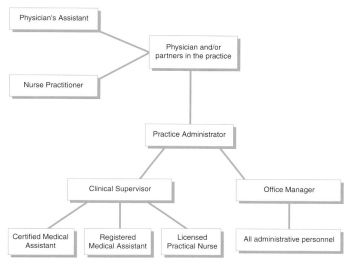

An organizational chart allows employees to identify their team members and see where they fit into the medical office team.

WORKPLACE DYNAMICS

The manner in which you and your coworkers interact is referred to as **workplace dynamics**. In an effective medical office, the workplace dynamics are strong and positive. Employees listen to each other, respect one another's opinions, and communicate messages professionally and honestly.

Communication with Patients

A trusting relationship with patients is built on honest and open communication. Most patients come to see the physician because they are not feeling well or because they are in pain. As a medical assistant, you should use the therapeutic communication skills that you've learned to help the patient identify his health problem and understand the physician's plan of treatment. Listening to and understanding the patient's concerns are key steps in the communication process. All communication with patients should be professional and respectful.

> Let your coworkers know you care.

Communication with Coworkers

Your communication with your coworkers should be polite, clear, and open. You should use effective listening techniques and provide feedback. Working in a medical office can be a challenge for everybody. Keep the workplace dynamics strong by communicating with support and compassion. A smile and a kind word to the receptionist during a busy day shows that you understand and care.

Communication with Supervisors

Your office supervisor is an important resource. You may need to speak with your office supervisor on many different occasions. As with all interactions, remember to keep the lines of communication open. Topics for discussion may include scheduling, policies and procedures, staffing, and workplace environment. Remember to address personal issues confidentially and respectfully.

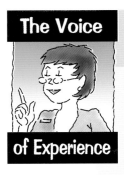

The Voice of Experience

WORKPLACE GOSSIP AND PATIENT CONFIDENTIALITY

Q: *How do I maintain patient confidentiality when socializing with coworkers?*

A: Office gossip is hard to avoid in any workplace, but it's very important to steer clear of situations where gossip might result in a breach of patient confidentiality. Ideally, gossip should be minimized or eliminated altogether in the workplace. However, if you must discuss a patient with a coworker, be sure keep your voices low and avoid talking about the patient by name. Never discuss patients' problems in public places where you might be overheard.

Send and Receive

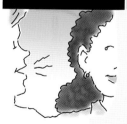

COMMUNICATION ROADBLOCKS

Let's say that you need to talk to your office manager about scheduling a few days off next month. Choosing the appropriate time to discuss this is critical. Let's look at an ineffective way and an effective way of handling this situation.

Ineffective:

- You approach the office manager, who is busy with another task. You interrupt her to say, "Hi, Sharon, I need to talk to you about scheduling a few days off next month."

- Sharon is too busy to acknowledge your request.

- You tap Sharon on the shoulder to get her attention. "Excuse me, Sharon. I need to schedule a few days off next month."

- Sharon stops what she is doing and says to you, "Can't you see that I'm busy? You'll have to talk to me about this later!"

There are two important errors in this situation. First, scheduling a few days off is not a high-priority issue. A better time to discuss scheduling would be before office hours. Or, you could request a time to talk with your office manager in a memo or an e-mail message. Let your manager suggest a convenient time. Second, it's always best to ask a coworker if she is busy before you bring up a new topic. Being respectful of others includes being considerate of their time. Let's look at this situation again.

Effective:

- You approach the office manager who is busy with another task. You wait until she seems to have a break before asking, "Excuse me, Sharon, I'm sorry to interrupt, but I need to talk with you about a scheduling issue I have for next month. When would be a good time to do that?"

- Sharon appreciates your polite and considerate request and responds, "No problem. I'm really busy now, but how about later on this afternoon at around 4?"

- You appreciate Sharon's willingness to talk so soon. "That would be great. Thanks!"

  Remember, being disrespectful, impolite, unclear, and unprofessional are all communication roadblocks that you should avoid.

Avoid communication roadblocks!

Communication with Physicians

The physicians at your office depend on you to share important information with them. Here is a list of tips to help you communicate effectively with the physicians at your office:

- *Be professional.* Address the physician as "Doctor." Use correct medical terms. Treat the physician with respect.

- *Prioritize.* Address important matters first. Learn to distinguish between information that must be discussed immediately and information that can wait.

- *Follow office procedures.* Your office has specific procedures to follow in emergency situations, urgent situations, and situations that need to be addressed in a timely manner. You should be aware of the resources that are available in your community for dealing with large-scale emergencies.

DISCIPLINARY ACTIONS

Disciplinary action usually results when an employee does not follow the office rules or policies. Some behaviors that require disciplinary action include coming in late too many times, leaving early often, not showing up for work, or not communicating effectively or appropriately with patients.

Every medical office has its own way of documenting disciplinary actions. An office may document verbal discussion or use specific disciplinary forms. The facts related to the action are listed on the form. The form should also include any expected changes in behavior. In some cases, disciplinary action may include additional training for the employee.

OFFICE MANAGERS AND OTHER COWORKERS

In the course of your day, you'll interact with your office manager many times. The office manager, or business manager, communicates with patients, physicians, and medical office

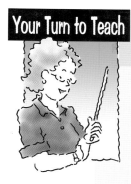

Your Turn to Teach

COMMUNITY RESOURCES FOR DEALING WITH LARGE-SCALE EMERGENCIES

As a member of the health care community, you should be aware of local resources for coping with large-scale emergencies. Such emergencies may include natural disasters, such as hurricanes, tornadoes, fires, or floods, or man-made disasters. In addition to resources provided by the federal government, local communities have developed their own resources for dealing with these types of emergency situations.

If patients ask where they can obtain information about local emergency management resources, the following agencies and offices can help them get started on their search:

- state and county government offices
- school districts
- fire departments
- local law enforcement agencies
- hospitals
- emergency medical services
- local chapters of aid organizations such as the American Red Cross and the Salvation Army
- local shelters

staff. He handles maintenance, inventory, scheduling, and staffing issues. If you have questions about office procedures or policies, ask your office manager!

As you can see, the office manager has a lot to do. Be supportive and respectful of his position by showing patience and courtesy. Your coworkers all work hard during the day. Supporting each other is critical. Some other ways to help keep communication strong among coworkers include:

- attending scheduled staff meetings
- using bulletin boards
- accessing the office intranet
- using e-mail
- using memos

Staff Meetings

Staff meetings help employees discuss important topics and issues. Staff meetings should be organized. They should follow an agenda, and a staff member should report and record the meeting minutes. Remember to address your personal concerns privately, not in a staff meeting.

Bulletin Boards

Using a bulletin board is an excellent way to post notices, policies, and procedures. The bulletin board should be placed in a central location where all employees can check it regularly. It's preferable that patients not see the employee bulletin board.

Office Intranet

Your office intranet is another useful tool for posting information about the medical practice and its employees. Check it often for important announcements or notices.

E-mail

Some offices provide a separate e-mail account for each employee. E-mail use should be limited to professional contacts only. Do not use your office e-mail account to send messages to family and friends. Also, do not use e-mail to discuss non–job-related issues.

Memos

A memo is a quick and easy way to provide a short message or reminder to an employee. Your office probably has a memo pad or memo forms to use. Keep a few in your pocket or on your desk. You can also use a computer to create a memo.

Managing Workplace Conflict

Even an outstanding health care team has to deal with occasional problems. When a conflict arises in your office, it's important that the problem be addressed in a timely manner. Conflict can make people uncomfortable, and they may not know how to manage it. Conflict can be managed by creating an environment where people can express and work through their differences in an atmosphere of respect.

WHAT IS CONFLICT?

Conflict results when a person feels that his needs, interests, or concerns are being threatened by another person or event. Conflict is not enjoyable, but it's a natural part of everyday life. It's a

Listen to This

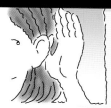

WORKPLACE DYNAMICS

Keeping workplace dynamics positive and effective can be a challenge. Here are some tips to keep in mind when interacting with your coworkers.

- Listen!
- Be aware of your own nonverbal communication.
- Use the employee bulletin board to post information about new policies or procedures.
- Arrive on time to staff meetings.
- Use the office intranet, e-mail, and memos to communicate with coworkers.
- Learn how to give and receive constructive criticism.

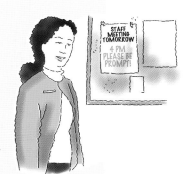

normal outcome of human interactions. You probably think of conflict as something negative. You may tend to think of conflict in terms of anger, hostility, violence, stress, and fear. People react to conflict in a variety of ways based on prior experiences. However, conflict does not have to be disruptive.

CAUSES AND SOURCES OF CONFLICT

Conflict can happen for many reasons. Often, people have different ways of handling a situation or addressing a problem. When people disagree with one another and express their different ideas, it creates a healthier workplace. It's important for all employees to know how to raise and address issues in the workplace.

Conflict can happen at work or in the home. There can be conflict between friends, family members, coworkers, or even strangers. The causes of conflict can be grouped into three categories. These categories are:

- communication differences
- personal differences
- structural differences

Not all differences create conflict. Remember, conflict only results when differences cause you to feel threatened.

Communication Differences

As you might guess, conflicts often occur because of something that is said, not said, or said ineffectively. Let's look at a simple example. Let's say you work with another medical assistant named Karen. On Tuesday, Karen would like to leave work a little early to go to an appointment. She asks you to restock the patient examination rooms for her, a duty for which she is usually responsible. If Karen communicates her need to you effectively, you'll likely restock the rooms and no conflict will occur.

But what if Karen communicates her need ineffectively? For example, what if Karen says to you as she is leaving, "Restock my rooms, okay? I have to leave. Thanks. Bye!" In this example, Karen's unexpected request fails to consider your needs. Because she failed to give you adequate notice about restocking the examination rooms, you may feel as if she is taking advantage of you.

In short, when messages are sent and received in an ineffective manner, communication differences occur. And when communication differences occur, conflict results.

Misunderstanding

Misunderstandings in communication are another source for conflict. For example, suppose a coworker asks you in the morning, "Could you restock the patient examination rooms this afternoon? I have to run out for a little while. Thanks!"

Your coworker makes it sound as though he will be back after a little while. But what if he ends up being gone the rest of the afternoon? Your understanding of his request ends up being very different from what happened. In this case, there is a misunderstanding between what was said and what was meant.

As you have learned, feedback is critical to effective communication. Always make sure that what you *think* you understand is what the other person meant.

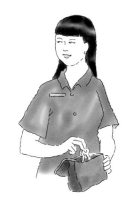

> Sure, I can restock the examination rooms while you go to your appointment. How long do you think it will take?

Poor Communication

Another way that conflict can happen is when a message is poorly communicated. Let's suppose a coworker stops you in the hallway and says, "Hey! I really need you to restock the patient examination rooms on Tuesday afternoon. Thanks!"

Your coworker dashes off assuming that you can restock the patient examination rooms. The problem in this example is that she never gives you time to respond to her request.

Differences in Communication Styles

Everybody has a different communication style. Most of the time, such differences make communicating more interesting! But, sometimes, these differences result in conflict. For example, suppose a coworker stops you in the hallway during a very busy morning and says, "Hey, I need you to restock the patient examination rooms on Tuesday afternoon. Thanks! I'll make it up to you!"

Your coworker's informal communication style is too unprofessional for a work-related request. Also, you would probably prefer being *asked* to do a favor, not *told*.

Perceiving Others' Words and Actions

Conflict can also arise when you perceive what somebody else says or does in a negative way. How you perceive any situation is guided by your background, education, and life experiences. These things are different for everybody. Therefore, people have different perceptions, which can result in conflict.

Remember, when your perception of a situation differs from somebody else's, being understanding and tolerant will help resolve conflicts.

Personal Differences

Personal differences are natural and expected. Most of the time, you and your coworkers are quick to handle personal differences effectively. But, occasionally, such differences may create conflict. Types of personal differences include:

- unique personality traits
- background, education, and life experience
- value systems and goals

Unique Personality Traits

You can't expect to be everybody's best friend all the time. This is true in your personal life as well as in your professional life. And, the more people on your health care team, the more likely it is that you'll have personality differences with at least one of your coworkers. Always keep in mind that conflicts resulting from personality differences are best handled with tolerance and understanding.

Background, Education, and Life Experience

The way you were raised may be very different from the way somebody else was raised. The schools you went to may have been very different from the schools your coworkers attended. Your life experiences may also be different from somebody else's. These differences shape who you are.

"There are more pronounced differences between the generations today than ever before," says Claire Raines, coauthor of *Generations at Work.* "That's simply because our world has changed so much in the last 50 to 80 years." These generational differences may impact workplace communication and create conflict. To an older employee, communication skills may mean formal writing and speaking. But to an employee in his twenties, communication may mean sending messages using e-mail or instant messaging.

Value Systems and Goals

Members of the health care team may have different goals. Although it's valuable to have differing views around the team table, if there is not a shared common view of how all the pieces fit together as a system, the resulting conflict can be unproductive. Too often, some of the players on a team only represent their own interests.

Structural Differences

Each workplace has a certain organizational structure. You know where your position is in the structure of your workplace. Conflict arises when the organizational structure does not function as you expect. If your needs and goals, based on the workplace structure, differ from a coworker's, conflict can result. Some types of structural differences include:

- needs and functions
- personal goals and motivation
- responsibilities
- availability of resources

Needs and Functions

As a medical assistant, you're part of a health care team. This team has specific needs and a particular function. Your understanding of those needs and function should be the same as your coworkers' understanding. If the health care team does not share a common view of its needs and function, conflict can result. Sometimes, these types of conflicts can be cleared up by referring to the practice's mission statement.

Personal Goals and Motivation

Your personal goals may be very different from somebody else's. In addition, what motivates you to meet those goals may not be what motivates another person. Like many of the other differences discussed in this section, this is natural. However, when coworkers have different goals and sources of motivation, conflict can result.

For example, for some individuals, the satisfied feeling of a job well done may be enough to motivate them to perform their daily tasks. But others may require a more concrete motivator, such as the promise of career advancement or a pay raise. Various sources of motivation can cause you and your coworkers to approach work in different ways, which sometimes leads to conflict.

Responsibilities

You and your coworkers share the same professional responsibility—to provide care for patients. But your personal responsibilities are probably very different from those of your coworkers'. For example, you may have young children to care for at home, whereas another coworker may not have children. Or you might have a personal conflict at home that makes it hard for you to focus at work. These kinds of situations can create conflict between coworkers.

Availability of Resources

The medical office can be a busy place. When employees have too many tasks to carry out or when they lack the necessary resources to carry out those tasks, conflict can result. For example, as a medical assistant, your tasks can vary from greeting patients in the reception area, retrieving and filing medical records, taking patients' vital signs, or preparing patients for minor office surgery. But suppose you were responsible for *all* of these tasks in a large medical practice. It would be impossible to meet the needs of every patient! You'd probably feel tired and stressed, which could lead to conflicts with your coworkers.

To keep these types of conflicts from arising, tasks and responsibilities should be distributed evenly among office employees. When each member of the health care team does her part, patients' needs can be met more effectively.

STAGES OF CONFLICT

Conflict usually occurs in certain stages. When you know how to recognize these stages, you can help resolve conflict before it escalates. Additionally, resolving conflict early is much easier than resolving conflict that has been going on for a long time.

Let's go through an example to help illustrate the stages of conflict.

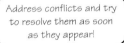

Address conflicts and try to resolve them as soon as they appear!

Need, Goal, or Desire Is Blocked

In the first stage of conflict, a need, goal, or desire is blocked by another person. For example, suppose that whenever you take a patient's blood pressure, you always place the blood pressure cuff back in a designated drawer in the examination room. You have even labeled the drawer to remind others to return the cuff to the proper place. That way, you and others always know where to find the blood pressure cuff. However, one of the other medical assistants, Sam, consistently forgets to put the blood pressure cuff back in this drawer after he uses it.

In this example, your goal of having an organized way of keeping track of the blood pressure cuff is being blocked by another medical assistant.

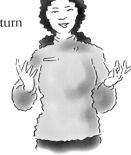

Frustration Sets In

In the next stage of conflict, you become frustrated at having your need, goal, or desire blocked. Let's return to the example of the blood pressure cuff. Suppose you have asked Sam on several different occasions to please return the cuff to the labeled drawer. Still, he forgets. This frustrates you because your attempts to remind Sam are ineffective. Sam is probably frustrated, too, because you keep nagging him!

Frustration Leads to Blame

In the next stage of conflict, frustration increases to the point where you blame another person for your feelings. For example, you might blame Sam for your frustration over the blood pressure cuff. You might say aloud or think to yourself, "I am so frustrated. And it's all Sam's fault!"

Anger Results

In the next stage of conflict, frustration becomes anger. When you're angry, you may do or say things that are unfair and negative. You may make broad statements based only on the frustrating situation. For example, you might say to Sam, "I can't work with you! You can't even remember to put the blood pressure cuff back in the right spot!"

Reaction to Anger

At the peak stage of a conflict, those involved react to each other with frustration and anger. This causes the conflict to increase.

Suppose you have tried again and again to get Sam to replace the blood pressure cuff. Then, late one afternoon, you're behind schedule. You go to take a patient's blood pressure only to find the cuff is not where it's supposed to be. You look everywhere and still cannot find it. This uses up valuable time. You fall further behind schedule. Finally, you end up having to interrupt Sam, who is with a patient, to get the blood pressure cuff from him. Later, you and Sam exchange angry words about the incident. You both react to each other's anger and frustration, causing the conflict to escalate.

Management Intervenes

The workplace is not the place for anger. When conflict reaches this stage, it's out of control. When this happens, an office manager, physician, or other coworker must step in to help resolve the conflict. She might schedule a meeting to discuss the issue. Or she might offer a solution that resolves the conflict immediately. For example, a physician might overhear your angry exchange with Sam. After hearing the details of the conflict, she might immediately suggest, "I have an idea. Let's order more blood pressure cuffs so each of you can have your own."

CONFLICT MANAGEMENT STYLES

There are many ways to manage conflict. Each management style has its own characteristics. Each style is effective in certain situations. The trick is learning to use the right management style for the right situation.

Win/Lose/Dominate

In the win/lose/dominate style of conflict management, one person's needs are emphasized over another person's needs. In other words, one person **dominates**, or takes over, the conflict. As a result, there is a winner and there is a loser. As you might guess, this style of conflict management should not be used all the time.

The win/lose/dominate style uses aggressive communication. Its main tool is forceful power. In an emergency, it provides quick, decisive action. For these reasons, this style of conflict management is most effective only in specific situations. For example, the win/lose/dominate style is most effective:

- in emergency situations when an immediate decision is necessary
- when unpopular actions need to be taken
- for resolving issues that are vital to an organization's welfare

For example, conflict may arise as a result of reducing the office budget, enforcing strict rules, or using disciplinary action against an employee for inappropriate behavior. In these situations, the win/lose/dominate style may be the best means of resolving the conflict.

Accommodating

In the accommodating style of conflict management, a person willingly gives up his needs for the needs of the other person. To **accommodate** means to allow for the wishes or needs of another person to be met. This method of conflict resolution is also known as "smoothing over." You might need to be accommodating to end or prevent conflict in the following situations:

- when you think you may be wrong
- to show how reasonable you are
- when an issue is more important to others than it is to you

The result of giving in or accommodating is that it minimizes your loss in a conflict when you're clearly outmatched or losing. It also helps subordinates grow by letting them make their own mistakes from which they can learn.

Compromise

In the compromise style of conflict management, each person forfeits something to gain something else. In other words, compromise includes making tradeoffs. In this type of resolution, each person's needs are considered equally. Compromise is often used to reach a temporary settlement to a complex issue. It's also used to solve conflict quickly. You might find that compromise is effective when your goal is important, but it's not worth the price of conflict.

For example, suppose you're a "morning person" and you think that your supervisor should schedule all office meetings prior to the start of the workday. However, your coworker prefers meeting at the end of the day. In this situation, you may suggest a compromise and ask that your supervisor alternate meeting times.

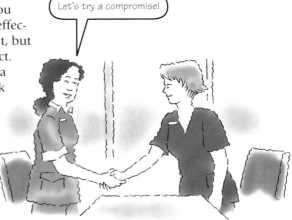

Let's try a compromise!

Avoidance

During **avoidance**, people ignore conflict. For example, you might suggest, "Perhaps if we do not bring it up, it will all blow over." Avoidance is a common response to the negative feelings associated with conflict.

With the avoidance approach, people's needs and concerns are not expressed. As a result, people are often confused about how to interact with one another. You might use avoidance when issues are trivial or when more important issues are pressing. Avoidance may give you time to cool down and gain perspective. Once time passes, you may be in a better position to resolve conflict. Or, you may use avoidance when you see no chance of things going your way.

Collaboration

Collaboration is blending individual needs and goals toward a larger common goal. This is also called "win-win problem solving." Collaboration results in a better solution than each individual could have achieved on his own. Collaboration is not easy, though. It requires assertive communication and cooperation.

Here are some situations when collaboration is effective:

- when an individual concern is too important to be dismissed
- to bring together differing insights or perspectives
- to gain long-term commitment by reaching a consensual agreement
- when individual feelings need to be addressed before an agreement can be reached

As you can see, collaboration takes time and effort from all persons involved. The reward is that each individual takes part in the solution. This helps build pride, self-worth, and confidence.

CONFLICT RESOLUTION IN COLLABORATIVE ENVIRONMENTS

As you have learned, conflict is natural. It can also be a healthy opportunity to grow and improve. But this can only happen when conflict resolution takes place in a setting that is positive and constructive. Here are some things to keep in mind when working to resolve any conflict.

- Conflict is natural.
- Resolutions are the result of open discussion.

- Resolutions should focus on issues, not the personalities of the people involved.
- Resolutions require those involved to be committed to search for alternatives.
- Resolutions are most effective when implemented right away.

Conflict Is Natural

Conflict is natural, but learning how to work through and resolve conflict is very important. Start any conflict resolution discussion with the reminder that you're committed to working through the conflict that has occurred.

Conflict can help you evaluate what's important and what isn't. It provides an opportunity to change the way you relate to other people and may help you improve who you are professionally and emotionally.

Open Discussion Resolves Conflict

Conflict can be resolved when all persons involved are willing to sit down and discuss the situation openly and honestly.

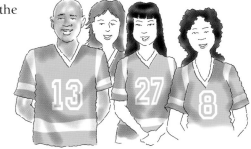

It's Not About You; It's About the Issue

Always keep words such as *I, you, me, we,* and *they* out of any resolution discussion. Keep discussions focused on the issues and not on the people involved.

All for One

Finding ways to resolve conflict can be tricky. Usually, there must be collaboration from one or all persons involved. It's vitally important that all parties involved in the process are committed to finding answers, compromises, or alternatives for resolving the conflict.

Working together as a team helps resolve conflict.

Conflict Resolution Now, Not Tomorrow

It's important that a resolution to a conflict goes into effect immediately. The sooner you begin using a resolution plan or agreement, the sooner the conflict will be resolved.

Supervisory Styles

Your manager is the person who oversees the employees at your medical office. One of your manager's goals is to identify your needs and the needs of your coworkers effectively. A good man-

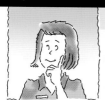

WHAT'S THE BEST WAY TO RESOLVE CONFLICT?

What if you have an ongoing conflict with someone you see at work every day? What's the best way to resolve the conflict?

The first step to resolve your conflict is to sit down with the other person and discuss the problem. Arrange a time and place where you're both comfortable, unthreatened, and where you will not be interrupted or distracted.

If you feel that you need a third person to help mediate the discussion, agree on who that person should be. Also, if the problem involves many coworkers, it might make more sense to call a special staff meeting to discuss and resolve the problem. In any case, remember to be respectful and considerate of one another's opinions and ideas. Be committed to finding a way to resolve the conflict. Remember, you're part of a health care team!

ager motivates employees by responding to their needs appropriately. Managers often use different management styles when supervising their employees. Three such styles are:

- authoritative management
- participative management
- servant-leadership

Let's talk about the characteristics of these management styles.

AUTHORITATIVE MANAGEMENT

The first type of management style is called **authoritative management**. With this style, the manager makes all decisions relating to the practice. Other employees do not take part in making decisions. This is also referred to as a *unilateral* style of management.

PARTICIPATIVE MANAGEMENT

Another type of management style is called **participative management**. With this style, the manager permits other employees to take part in decision making. In other words, employees are allowed to participate in the management of the practice. The participative management style also gives employees a certain

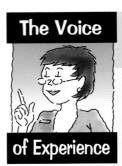

WORKING WITH THE SERVANT-LEADERSHIP MANAGEMENT STYLE

Q: *What is a servant-leader?*

A: Servant-leadership emphasizes the importance of service to others, a sense of community, and sharing decision-making power. The servant-leader is an employee who is a servant first and a leader second. An employee serves others by helping them become healthier, wiser, freer, and more independent.

amount of independence in performing their routine work activities.

SERVANT-LEADERSHIP

A third type of management style is called **servant-leadership.** This term was coined and defined by management expert Robert Greenleaf in 1970. The servant-leadership approach to management emphasizes service before leadership. Managers serve the people they lead. They help their employees grow and improve so that they can become more effective workers. Managers also carry out the decisions and wishes of their employees for the greater good of the organization.

Employment Communication Skills

In addition to communicating with patients and coworkers, a professional medical assistant must develop skills for communicating about employment. These skills include:

- developing a resume
- writing a cover letter
- preparing for an interview

RESUME

A **resume** is a brief summary of your work experience and professional qualifications. These facts can help others decide if you're an appropriate candidate for a specific job. Resumes create a first impression, so it's vital that they are accurate and error-free.

You can use one of several different styles to create a resume. These styles include:

- standard resume
- chronological resume
- functional resume
- combination resume

Writing a resume is not difficult. Simply choose the style that best suits the job for which you're applying. Follow the organizational details of that style to create a neat and professional resume.

Standard Resume

A **standard resume** organizes information into separate categories. These categories may include:

- personal information
- job objective
- work experience
- education
- work skills

This kind of resume can also include categories for memberships, honors, and any special skills or interests related to the job.

Chronological Resume

A **chronological resume** lists important information by date. For example, in listing your work experience, you would start with your most recent place of employment (including the date) and move backward.

Functional Resume

A **functional resume** includes a series of paragraphs that identify a candidate's most important work skills. List these paragraphs in order from most pertinent to the job applied for to least pertinent.

Combination Resume

A **combination resume** combines the chronological and functional resume styles. This resume arranges information in paragraphs. It also shows work experiences in chronological order with the most recent date first.

COVER LETTER

A **cover letter** is a letter that accompanies a resume. It should be clear and concise while showcasing your qualifications.

Tina Elmwood C.M.A.
22 Brandy Drive
Dayton, Ohio 00000
444-777-6666

Employment Objective: To use my medical assisting skills in a challenging position. My goal is to work with children. (*Change this sentence to reflect the type of office that you are applying to.*)

Experience:

Externship (160 hours) at Family Practice Associates, Bayview Drive, Dayton, Ohio (*If you have a positive evaluation from your preceptor, bring it with you to the interview. Do not attach it to the resume.*)

Education:

Medical Assisting Program, Diploma. Graduated June 2008. West County Community College, Dayton Ohio (*Bring a copy of your diploma and transcripts to the interview. Do not attach them unless employer has specifically requested them.*)
Dayton High School, Diploma. Graduated June 2006. Dayton, Ohio

Skills:

Clinical and Laboratory skills listed on Role Delineation for Medical Assisting

Administrative skills listed on Role Delineation for Medical Assisting

Comfortable using all types of standard office equipment

Familiar with XYZ software programs (*List software programs that you are comfortable with. If you know what type of software the office uses, list that as well.*)

Certifications:

Certified Medical Assistant, American Association of Medical Assistants (*Bring copy to interview or attach to résumé.*)
Cardiopulmonary Resuscitation, American Heart Association (*Bring copy to interview or attach to résumé.*)

References available upon request.

A functional resume works well for recent graduates because it focuses on the candidate's skills and qualifications rather than employment history.

The information included in your cover letter should be brief but meaningful. The purpose of the cover letter is to impress the reader enough to want to interview you. A standard cover letter includes three paragraphs:

- opening paragraph
- middle paragraph
- closing paragraph

Opening Paragraph

In the opening paragraph, state the reason for the cover letter. State the name of the health care position for which you're applying. Also, describe how you learned about the job opening.

Middle Paragraph

In the middle paragraph, state why you're interested in working for the medical organization. Describe why you want to do this

Beatrice Meza C.M.A.
123 Main Street
West Harford, CT 00000
888-999-6666

Employment Objective: To use my medical assisting skills in a challenging position. My goal is to work in an obstetrical office. (*Change this sentence to reflect the type of office that you are applying to.*)

Education:

2007–2008 Medical Assisting Program; Mountain Laurel Community College, West Hartford, Connecticut (*Bring a copy of your diploma and transcripts to the interview. Do not attach them unless employer has specifically requested them.*)

Externship:

July 2008–(160 hours) Women's Health Care Center, Hartford, Connecticut (*If you have a positive evaluation from your preceptor, bring it with you to the interview. Do not attach it to the résumé.*)

Work Experience:

July 2007–present Receptionist, Dermatology Consultants, West Hartford, Connecticut. Worked part time while I was in school. Answered and triaged telephone calls. Assisted with various other medical administrative responsibilities. (*If you have a reference letter from this employer, bring it with you to the interview. Be prepared to answer questions about why you are leaving this position.*)
May 2004–July 2007 Cashier/Clerk for SuperMarket Grocers, West Hartford, Connecticut. Worked part time. Responsible for training new employees. Promoted to senior cashier.

Skills:

Clinical and Laboratory skills listed on the Role Delineation for Medical Assisting
Administrative skills listed on the Role Delineation for Medical Assisting
Comfortable using all types of standard office equipment
Familiar with XYZ software programs (*List software programs that you are comfortable with. If you know what type of software the office uses, list that as well.*)

Activities/Honors

Student Government representative
Most Improved Medical Assisting Student in 2007

References available upon request.

A chronological resume is particularly useful if your employment history is relevant to the position you're seeking.

type of work. For example, for a job in a pediatrician's office, you might write, "My goal is to play a role in improving the health of children."

Also include a brief summary of your qualifications, achievements, and any training that qualifies you for the position.

Closing Paragraph

In the closing paragraph, refer to your enclosed resume and encourage positive action. For example, you may write, "I look forward to speaking with you soon." You may also request an interview by saying, "I would appreciate the opportunity to further discuss my candidacy in an interview."

INTERVIEW SKILLS

It takes time and effort to develop good interview skills. However, good interview skills are critical to being hired for a job. In many hiring situations, the candidate who gives the best interview is hired for the job.

Know the Health Care Facility

It's important to be as prepared as possible for an interview. As part of your preparation, find out as much as you can about the health care facility to which you applied. For example, research the services and procedures the facility provides. Think of questions you might ask about the facility's operations.

> Prepare for your interview by being organized.

Be Organized

Create a folder for your interview. In it, include all the materials you'll need for the health care interview. Here's what your interview folder should contain:

- a copy of your resume
- a copy of your cover letter
- a list of personal and professional references
- a completed employment application

It's also a good idea to bring a notepad and pen or pencil. That way you can jot down questions or notes during the interview.

Prepare to Answer Questions

Part of being prepared for an interview is having an idea of the types of questions you might be asked. The following is a list of typical interview questions:

- What are your strengths?
- What are your weaknesses?
- Why do you want this position?
- What are your goals?
- Why did you leave your last position?
- Do you work better alone or as a member of a team?

Think about how you would answer each of these questions. Make sure your answers to these and other interview questions are positive and confident. Remember to be aware of nonverbal messages during an interview.

A good way to practice your interview skills is to have friends or family members play the part of a potential employer and ask you typical interview questions.

Prepare to Ask Questions

After the interviewer asks you questions, you'll most likely be asked, "Do you have any questions?" Refer to your notepad for any questions you wrote down during the interview. Here are some questions you might consider asking during an interview:

- What is the job description for this position?
- If it's not personal, why is the current employee leaving?
- What are the opportunities for future advancement?
- How long is the training or probation period?
- What kind of job performance or evaluation process is there?
- What is the benefits package? Is there a 401(k) or other retirement plan offered? Is life or health insurance included in the benefits package?
- Is time off provided for skill improvement or continuing education?

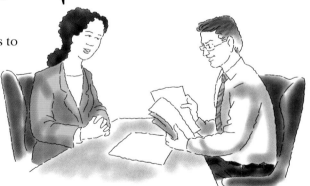

Nonverbal communication, including good posture, eye contact, and a relaxed, friendly manner, are essential to a good interview.

Sell Yourself!

The goal of any interviewer is to hire the person who will make the most positive contribution to the workplace. Your goal is to show the interviewer that you're the best person for the job. Make sure you emphasize your strengths during the interview.

Communication and Professional Growth

You have learned many ways to use your communication skills to display confidence, inner strength, and knowledge. You know that your communication with patients and coworkers should

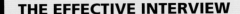

Listen to This   THE EFFECTIVE INTERVIEW

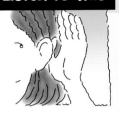

Here's a quick list of reminders to help you get through any interview with flying colors!

- Speak clearly and distinctly.
- Dress appropriately and professionally.
- Arrive on time or a few minutes early.
- Offer your hand to shake the interviewer's hand.
- Make eye contact when the interviewer speaks.
- Be courteous and diplomatic.
- Be attentive, listen, and learn.

promote good health and well-being. Developing good communication skills helps you grow as a professional.

YOU AND YOUR PERSONAL LIFE

You also know that it's important to always be professional in the workplace. However, professionalism does not end when you go home for the day. Your interactions with strangers, friends, and family members should display the same positive qualities you show when you're working. Extending positive qualities to other aspects of your life will help you grow as a person.

YOU AND THE COMMUNITY

You can also grow as a professional by going the extra mile to promote your occupation at the community level. You can do this by participating in community activities connected to your professional organization. You can also participate in promoting healthy lifestyles within your community.

YOU AND YOUR COWORKERS

As a professional, remember to respect all members of your health care team. Understand the importance of individual roles in your workplace. Learning to work together with mutual respect and consideration promotes professional growth. It also makes the whole team stronger and more effective.

YOU AND YOUR CAREER

You'll continue to grow as a professional throughout your career. Learn from every challenge. Find something positive in every interaction. In addition, continue to develop and improve your communication skills. By doing so, you ensure that your career as a medical assistant will be as rewarding as possible.

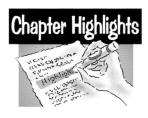

Chapter Highlights

- Effective communication with all members of the health care team requires professionalism, courtesy, honesty, integrity, and confidentiality. It also follows a code of ethics.

- Workplace dynamics involve the manner in which coworkers interact. These dynamics must be positive and professional to keep the office running smoothly.

- Conflict is a disagreement that results when a person feels that his needs, interests, or concerns are being threatened by another person.

- Sources of conflict include communication differences, personal differences, and structural differences.

- In the first stage of a conflict, a need, goal, or desire is blocked. The stages that follow include frustration, blame, anger, and reactions to anger.

- In the win/lose/dominate style of conflict management, one person gains and one person loses. In the accommodating style, one person gives in to another person's needs. In the compromise style, both people make tradeoffs. In avoidance, the conflict is ignored.

- In authoritative management, the manager makes all decisions. In participative management, employees contribute to decision making. In servant-leadership, managers serve the people they lead and carry out decisions for the improvement of the organization.

- Developing a resume involves choosing an appropriate style and following organizational details to create a neat and professional summary of your professional qualifications.

- Techniques for a successful interview include researching the health care facility to which you applied, being organized, anticipating questions you'll be asked, preparing questions to ask, and being able to sell yourself.

- Developing and practicing therapeutic communication skills helps medical assistants grow professionally and personally.

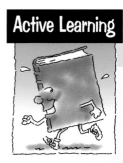

Active Learning

HONE YOUR PROFESSIONAL COMMUNICATION SKILLS

Complete one of the following tasks to help strengthen your professional communication skills:

- Prepare a resume.
- Write a cover letter.
- Research the code of ethics for your profession. Write a paragraph explaining how this code influences communications in the medical office.
- Determine your usual conflict management style and write a paragraph describing how you used it to resolve a recent conflict.

INTERVIEW PRACTICE

Practice your job interviewing skills with a partner. Have one person pose as the interviewer and ask each of the typical interview questions below:

- What are your strengths?
- What are your weaknesses?
- Why do you want this position?
- What are your goals?
- Why did you leave your last position?
- Do you work better alone or as a member of a team?

Then, switch roles and repeat the exercise. Which questions were most difficult to answer? Discuss your responses with your partner.

GLOSSARY

abuse   the purposeful act of hurting another person; can be the result of something that is done to another person, or something vital that is withheld, such as food [Chapter 6]

acceptance stage   the final stage of grief in which a patient becomes calm and accepting and willingly decides to deal with the reality of her loss [Chapter 6]

accommodate   allow for the wishes or needs of another person to be met [Chapter 9]

active exercise   a form of exercise in which people move their bodies by themselves [Chapter 7]

addiction   a disease in which a person craves something such as alcohol or drugs and acts on those cravings, even when such action is harmful to that person or to others [Chapter 6]

address book   a feature of e-mail software that includes a collection of e-mail addresses [Chapter 8]

adolescence   a period of rapid growth and development that occurs between childhood and adulthood [Chapter 3]

advance directive   a statement of a patient's wishes regarding health care prior to a critical medical event [Chapter 4]

agenda   a brief outline of the topics to be discussed at a meeting [Chapter 8]

AIDS (acquired immunodeficiency syndrome)   an incurable disease caused by the virus HIV (human immuno-deficiency virus) that specifically targets a person's immune system [Chapter 6]

anger   a strong feeling of displeasure or unhappiness that is often antagonistic in nature [Chapter 6]

anger stage   a stage of grief in which a person may experience rage, hostility, and emotional instability [Chapter 6]

anxiety   an emotional state, which may or may not be based on reality, in which a person feels uneasy, apprehensive, or fearful [Chapter 6]

attachment   a file (such as a document or photo) that is sent along with an e-mail message [Chapter 8]

authoritative management a supervisory style in which the manager makes all decisions [Chapter 9]

autonomy independence [Chapter 3]

avoidance a conflict management style in which people ignore conflict [Chapter 9]

bargaining stage one of the stages of grief; the person wants to "make a deal" with someone he feels has control over his fate, such as God or a health care provider [Chapter 6]

bias an opinion that favors one thing over another, often unfairly or without basis in fact or reason; prejudice [Chapter 5]

bilingual able to speak and understand two languages [Chapter 5]

block format a format for professional letters in which all lines are flush left and not indented [Chapter 8]

body language a form of nonverbal communication that involves an exchange of messages without using words [Chapter 4]

chain of command a series of positions within the organizational structure that are organized according to level of authority [Chapter 9]

child abuse any harmful behavior toward or mistreatment of a child [Chapter 6]

chronological resume a type of resume format in which important information is listed in order by date [Chapter 9]

clarification the act of making something clearer and easier to understand [Chapter 5]

closed-ended questions questions that are asked to gather specific information from a patient and can be answered with a word or phrase [Chapter 4]

cognitive relating to the ability to think and reason logically and to learn new ideas [Chapter 3]

combination resume a type of resume format that combines the chronological and functional resume styles; information is arranged in paragraphs, and work experience is listed in chronological order with the most recent date stated first [Chapter 9]

compensation a defense mechanism in which a person attempts to make up for a real or imagined weakness or deficiency [Chapter 4]

computer virus a program that can invade a computer and destroy files [Chapter 8]

confidentiality respecting privileged information that is held within a protected relationship, such as the relationship between patient and physician [Chapter 4]

conflict   discord resulting from differences between people; occurs when a person feels that another person or event threatens their needs, interests, or concerns [Chapter 9]

congruent message   a message in which the content and process of the message agree [Chapter 2]

conscience   a person's inner understanding of right and wrong [Chapter 3]

consultation   a request for the opinion of another physician [Chapter 7]

context   the situation in which messages are delivered and received, which in turn influences the outcome of any communications [Chapter 2]

continuous reinforcement   a response to a specific behavior in which that behavior is reinforced every time it happens [Chapter 3]

coping mechanism   a way of lessening the negative effects of stress or a stressor [Chapter 7]

cover letter   a letter that accompanies a resume [Chapter 9]

criminal violence   any violence that breaks a law; examples include stalking, physical abuse, and sexual abuse [Chapter 6]

crises   psychosocial dilemmas that must be mastered in order to for a person to grow and develop [Chapter 3]

cue detection   the ability to sense a patient's nonverbal cues, which is essential to effective communication [Chapter 3]

cultural competence   the set of beliefs, skills, and attitudes that can be used to interact effectively with patients of all cultures [Chapter 5]

culture   the set of learned and shared beliefs, values, and expectations that people use in their social interactions with others [Chapter 5]

defense mechanisms   conscious or unconscious mental tools that people use to cope with their feelings [Chapter 4]

denial   a defense mechanism in which a person fails to acknowledge a problem, an experience, or a reality [Chapter 4]

denial stage   a stage of grief in which the patient chooses not to accept that a loss will or has happened [Chapter 6]

depression   a feeling of extreme sadness or hopelessness that can be caused by external events such as the loss of a loved one, a sudden traumatic event, the loss of a job, or by an internal event, such as the imbalance of certain chemicals in the brain [Chapter 6]

depression stage   a stage of grief in which the patient goes through extreme feelings of sadness and hopelessness [Chapter 6]

dignity the state of being worthy [Chapter 3]

disability any condition that restricts a person's major life activities and functions [Chapter 6]

displacement a defense mechanism in which a person shifts the angry emotion of a situation from a threatening to a non-threatening object [Chapter 4]

diversity the variety of attitudes and beliefs found in a society that consists of many different cultures and groups [Chapter 5]

domestic violence the abuse of one family member by another [Chapter 6]

dominate take over [Chapter 9]

ego a force behind human nature that is more aware of the world around it than the id is; is able to navigate life's obstacles to satisfy the id's desires [Chapter 3]

ego ideal a person's understanding of the self, formed in childhood, based on rewards and positive models [Chapter 3]

ego identity a person's understanding of himself and how he fits in with the rest of society [Chapter 3]

ego integrity a person's ability to reflect on the course of her life, including the choices that she has made, and to come to terms with life as she has lived it; often associated with wisdom [Chapter 3]

elder abuse the abuse or neglect of an older person [Chapter 6]

e-mail electronic messages sent through a computer network [Chapter 8]

empathy the ability to identify with another person's world, experience, or situation [Chapter 1]

epigenetic principle a principle that states that development occurs as a personality unfolds following a preset plan [Chapter 3]

exercise any activity that uses muscles voluntarily or involuntarily to maintain fitness [Chapter 7]

facsimile (fax) machine a communications device that can send and receive printed material over a phone line [Chapter 8]

feedback responses and reactions received from others [Chapter 1]

functional resume a type of resume format that includes a series of paragraphs that identify a candidate's most important work skills [Chapter 9]

generativity a person's concern for the next generation and all future generations [Chapter 3]

geriatric relating to the branch of medicine that deals specifically with older adult patients [Chapter 3]

harassment   any annoying or stressful comment or behavior that is known to be unwelcome [Chapter 6]

hardware   the equipment and machinery that make up the computer, including the CPU (central processing unit), keyboard, monitor, and hard drive [Chapter 8]

Health Insurance Portability and Accountability Act of 1996 (HIPAA)   a federal law that set standards for the protection of private patient information and for submitting claims to health insurance companies [Chapter 4]

health maintenance   preventing diseases and staying as healthy as possible at all times [Chapter 7]

hierarchy of needs   a pyramid of human needs developed by Abraham Maslow that states that certain needs are more basic than others, and that these needs must be met before an individual can concentrate on higher-level needs [Chapter 1]

HIV (human immunodeficiency virus)   a virus transmitted via blood and other body fluids that targets the human immune system; people with HIV can go on to develop AIDS (acquired immunodeficiency syndrome) [Chapter 6]

holistic   an adjective used to describe care of the whole person, physically and emotionally [Chapter 3]

id   a force behind human nature that represents the basic animal nature of a person and includes her most primal drives and instincts [Chapter 3]

identification   a defense mechanism in which a person unconsciously copies another person's behavior [Chapter 4]

impairment   any condition that weakens or lessens the effectiveness of something else [Chapter 6]

incongruent message   a message in which the content and process of the message disagree [Chapter 2]

indirect statements   statements that are used to obtain a response from a patient without making the patient feel that he is being questioned [Chapter 4]

informed consent   a statement of approval from a patient, often given in writing, to perform a given procedure after the patient has been educated about its benefits and risks [Chapter 4]

initiative   a positive response to challenges in which a person assumes responsibilities, learns new skills, and feels purposeful [Chapter 3]

instinct   an automatic, natural behavior that does not have to be thought about [Chapter 3]

interdisciplinary communication   the interaction between professionals from two or more medical specialties to meet a specific goal [Chapter 9]

intermittent reinforcement   a response to a specific behavior in which that behavior is reinforced only at certain intervals [Chapter 3]

Internet   global system used to connect one computer to another for the purpose of communication [Chapter 8]

intimacy   the ability to be close to others and to participate in society [Chapter 3]

intranet   a private network of computers that share data [Chapter 8]

isolation   the removal of oneself from love, friendship, and community [Chapter 3]

kinesics   the study of body movements and facial expressions as a form of nonverbal communication [Chapter 2]

linguistic competence   the ability to communicate effectively with all patients, including those who speak different languages [Chapter 5]

memorandum   a note or letter used for communication within the office or between departments [Chapter 8]

message   any thought or idea that is transmitted from one person to another [Chapter 2]

modem   a communication device that is used to connect a computer to the Internet [Chapter 8]

modified block format   a format for professional letters in which the date, subject line, closing, and signature are aligned at the center or to the right of center; all other lines are flush left [Chapter 8]

modified semiblock format   a format for professional letters in which the first sentence of each paragraph is indented five spaces, or tabbed once; the date, subject line, closing, and signature are aligned at the center or to the right of center [Chapter 8]

mutuality   a principle developed by Erik Erikson that refers to the interaction of multiple generations; the general pattern of interconnectedness across generations [Chapter 3]

narrative   a paragraph indicating the contact with the patient, what was done for the patient, and the outcome of any action [Chapter 8]

negative stress   stress that makes a person tense, anxious, angry, or depressed [Chapter 7]

neglect   a form of abuse in which a person fails to provide basic necessities for another dependent person in her care [Chapter 6]

nonverbal communication skills   the skills a person uses when employing body language, facial expressions, or physical gestures to communicate with others [Chapter 1]

notice of privacy practices   a written document, required by federal law, which is prominently displayed and gives the details of a health care provider's privacy practices [Chapter 4]

nutrition   the science of food and how different foods affect a person's health [Chapter 7]

open-ended questions   questions that can't be answered by a simple yes or no and invite a more personalized response [Chapter 2]

operant conditioning   modifications of a person's actions that occur when he encounters different stimuli that either reinforce or discourage his normal behavior [Chapter 3]

organizational structure   a hierarchical arrangement that specifies where each employee fits into the team [Chapter 9]

participative management   supervisory style in which the manager permits other employees to take part in decision making for the team [Chapter 9]

passive exercise   a form of exercise in which a therapist, nurse, or caregiver helps a person move each joint through its range of motion [Chapter 7]

pediatric   relating to the branch of medicine that deals specifically with infants, children, and adolescents [Chapter 3]

peripherals   things that are connected to or plugged into the basic computer system from the outside, such as the mouse, scanner, and printer [Chapter 8]

personal space   the comfortable physical distance that people maintain between themselves and others [Chapter 2]

pleasure principle   the drive to decrease pain and increase pleasure that is often associated with the id [Chapter 3]

positive stress   stress that allows a person to perform at peak levels and then relax afterward [Chapter 7]

problem-oriented medical record (POMR)   a common method of compiling information that lists each problem of the patient, usually at the beginning of the folder, and references each problem with a number throughout the folder [Chapter 8]

projection   a defense mechanism in which a person attributes her own thoughts to another individual [Chapter 4]

protected health information   data about a patient's past, present, or future medical treatment that contain one or more patient identifiers and are therefore confidential [Chapter 4]

rationalization   a way of justifying one's behavior [Chapter 4]

reality principle   a drive generally associated with the ego that strives to fulfill a need as soon as an appropriate pathway or object is found [Chapter 3]

receiver   the person who receives and interprets a sender's message [Chapter 2]

referral the process of sending or guiding someone to another source (such as a medical specialist) for assistance [Chapter 7]

regression a defense mechanism that involves going back to an earlier stage of development during periods of high stress [Chapter 4]

repression a defense mechanism that uses forgetting or "temporary amnesia" as a way of dealing with an upsetting or traumatic experience [Chapter 4]

respect a person's ability to communicate sincerely that he believes in another person's worth and dignity [Chapter 1]

resume document summarizing an individual's work experience or professional qualifications [Chapter 9]

salutation an introductory phrase that greets the reader of a letter [Chapter 8]

self-actualization the state of mind in which one's basic needs are satisfied and a person is able to take full responsibility for her own life; also, the final stage of a person's development in which her full potential is finally realized [Chapter 1]

self-concept the mental image or picture a person has of himself [Chapter 1]

sender the person who sends the first message in a communication [Chapter 2]

servant-leadership supervisory style in which managers serve the people they lead; managers carry out the decisions and wishes of their employees for the greater good of the organization [Chapter 9]

SOAP a style of charting that includes subjective, objective, assessment, and planning notes [Chapter 8]

software application programs that direct the computer hardware to perform given tasks [Chapter 8]

spousal abuse the abuse or neglect of a spouse or other domestic partner [Chapter 6]

stagnation a state of being self-absorbed and obsessed with one's own needs [Chapter 3]

standard resume a type of resume format in which information is organized into separate categories, such as job objective, work experience, and education [Chapter 9]

stereotyping having an opinion of a certain culture, race, religion, age group, or other group that is based on negative or oversimplified views [Chapter 5]

stress a normal human response that occurs when a change in a person's environment is felt as a challenge, threat, or danger [Chapter 6]; the mind and body's response or reaction to a real or imagined threat, event, or change [Chapter 7]

stressor anything that causes a person to experience stress [Chapter 7]

sublimation a defense mechanism that involves directing a socially unacceptable impulse into a socially acceptable behavior [Chapter 4]

superego a force behind human nature that represents ideal behaviors and strives to be perfect rather than trying to be real or to achieve pleasure [Chapter 3]

sympathy the feeling of having pity for someone [Chapter 4]

teletypewriter (TTY) a special machine that allows communication on a phone with a hearing-impaired person [Chapter 8]

territoriality a person's urge to claim certain spaces as her own [Chapter 2]

undoing a defense mechanism in which a person tries to cancel a negative behavior as a way of making amends for something that was thought, said, or done [Chapter 4]

verbal communication skills the skills a person uses when employing written or spoken words to communicate with others [Chapter 1]

visualization a relaxation technique in which people allow their minds to wander and imagine freely [Chapter 7]

vocal paralanguage the extra clues in a person's voice, including tone, quality, volume, pitch, and range, that add meaning and emphasis to a message [Chapter 2]

workplace dynamics the manner in which coworkers interact with one another [Chapter 9]

INDEX

Page numbers in *italics* denote figures; page numbers followed by *t* denote tables.

A

Abbreviations, 256–257
Abuse
    of patients, 199–205
    substance, 167–171
    therapeutic techniques, 204
Acceptance
    grief and, 174
    parental, 7–8
Accuracy, in writing, 247
Acquired immune deficiency syndrome (AIDS), 161, 179–183
Active exercise, 225
Active listening, 45, 46, 48, 100
Adaptation
    to cultures, 136–137
    of style, 167
Addiction, 167–171
Adolescents, 76–81. *see also* children
Adult communication, 81–84
Adulthood, 81–82
Advance directives, 91, 119–120
Advising patients, 49–50, 111
African-American cultural factors, 145
African-Americans, risk factors in, 161
Age. *see also* children; older patients
    of adolescence, 76
    communication and, 69–72, 71–72
    culture and, 150
Agendas, 253
Aggression, 185–190
AIDS. *see* acquired immune deficiency syndrome (AIDS)
Alcoholism, 167–171
Anal stage of development, 59
Anemia, sickle-cell, 161
Anger
    causes of, 186

    consequences of, 190
    fear and, 191
    grief and, 173
    managing, 187
    as natural, 185–187
    recognizing, 187–188
    source of, 189
    therapeutic techniques, 188–190
    triggers of, 189–190
Anger displacement, 113
Anxiety, 183–185
Appetite, depression and, 196
Appointment reminders, 230–231
Appointments, missed, 234
Artificial limbs, 192
Asian cultural factors, 145–146
Atmosphere
    culturally diverse, 153
    positive, 16–18
    self-esteem and, 16–18
    work, 18
Attention, listening and, 43
Attitude
    culture and, 135
    verbal communication and, 37
Authenticity, 23
Authoritative management, 291
Autonomy *vs.* shame, 62
Avoidance, 289

B

Bargaining, grief and, 173–174
Beans, 221
Behavior, communication and, 54–55
Behavior modeling, 11–12
Behavioral learning theories, 67–68
Belief systems, 134–135
Beliefs, 134
Belonging, as need, 20

Bereavement, 150, 171–179
Bias, culture and, 153, 156–157
BID, 257t
Bilingual staff, 155–156
Biological development factors, 55
Blindness, 191–192, 192–193
BM, 257t
Body
    culture and, 142–143
    stress and, 213–214
Body image, 3
Body language. *see* nonverbal com-
    munication
Body weight, exercise and, 224
Breakdown, communication, 28–29
Breast cancer, 161
Breathing, deep, 186
Broad openings, 49
Brochures, 267–269
BRP, 257t
Business letter, 247–252, *250*

C

Cancellations, 235
Cancer, breast, 161
Cap, 257t
Capitalization, 246
Caring, 23
Caucasian cultural factors, 144
Challenges, 166–167
Changing subject, 50, 112
Channels of communication, 31–32
Chatting
    with adolescents, 77–81
    with children, 73–76
Chief complaint, 103
Child abuse, 202
Childhood, self-concept in, 4
Children. *see also* adolescents
    autonomy in, 63
    chatting with, 73–76
    effective communication with,
        73–76
    with illnesses, 73
    injections and, 76
    listening to, 75
    relationship with, 75
Choice, adolescents and, 78–79
Circular, self-concept and, 14–15
Circulation, 224–225
Clarification, 38, 138
Clarity, 34
Clichés, 50–51, 111

Closed-ended questions, 104
Cognitive development learning
    theory, 55–56
Cognitive impairments, 110–111
Collaboration, conflict management
    through, 289
Collaboration, with adults, 83–84
Colon (punctuation), 244–245
Comma, 245
Communication
    benefits of, 28
    breakdown, 28–29
    challenges, 166–167
    channels, 31–32
    cycle, 30–33
    importance of, 27–28
    nonverbal, 9
    reactions and responses in,
        14–16
    respect and, 10
    scope of, 27–29
    self-awareness and, 2
    self-esteem and, 9
    verbal, 9
Communication techniques, 72–73
Community resources, 209–211,
    236–237
Compassion, 170
Compensation for weakness, 113
Competency
    cultural, 133, 152–156
    interpersonal skills and, 23
    linguistic, 137–138
    self-esteem and, 7
Completeness, 34
Components, of self-concept, 6–7
Compromise, 289
Computers, 258–264
Concentration, depression and, 197
Concern, of patients, 47
Conciseness, 34
Concrete answers, 12
Concrete operational thought, 56
Conditioning, operant, 68–69, 70
Confidence, verbal communication
    and, 37
Confidentiality, 45, 78, 121
Conflict, management, 287–289
Conflict, resolution, 289–290
Conflict, stages of, 285–287
Conflict, workplace, 280–285
Conflict evaluation, 151
Congruent messages, 41–42
Connections with others, 8–9

Conscience, 58
Consent, 120–121, 181–182
Consistency
    feedback and, 16
    of message, 34
Consultations, 235
Context, 33–34
Continuous reinforcement, 68
Contradicting, 112
Control, in older adults, 87–89
Coping mechanisms, 214–216
Courtesy, 34
Cover letter, 293–295
Covey, Stephen, 22
Coworkers, 278–280
Criminal violence, 201
Criticism, 111, 188
Crying, 197
Cue detection, in elderly patients, 90
Culture
    adaptation and, 136–137
    African-American, 145
    age and, 150
    Asian, 145–146
    attitudes and, 135
    beliefs, 134–135
    body and, 142–143
    Caucasian, 144
    characteristics of, 132–133
    communication style and,
        155–156
    competence, 133, 135–137,
        152–156
    courtesy and, 143
    critical factors, 133–135
    definition of, 132
    diet and, 140, 141
    differences in, 136
    folk healers and, 143
    grief and, 150
    as guidebook, 138–152
    Hawaiian, 148–149
    health beliefs and, 140–150
    health needs and, 134
    Hispanic, 146–147
    judgment and, 153
    language and, 137–138
    learning about, 136
    medication and, 140–141
    Native American, 147–148
    outcomes and, 160–161
    patients and, 150–152
    policies and procedures and,
        152–153
    Puerto Rican, 147
    ritual and, 143
    self and, 135–136
    stereotypes and, 156–157
    traditions and, 134
Customs, cultural, 143
Cycle, communication, 30–33

D

DC, 257t
Deaf patients, 107–110, 265–267
Death
    clichés about, 50–51
    preparing for, 151
    reactions to, 171–179
Decision-making, grief and, 176–177
Deep breathing, 186
Defense mechanisms, 112–114
Defensiveness, 50
Delays, physician, 234
Delivery style, 82–83
Denial
    as defense mechanism, 112
    grief and, 173
Depression
    characteristics of, 194
    definition of, 194
    grief and, 174
    signs of, 194–197
    suicide and, 198–199
    therapeutic techniques, 197–198
Despair, 65–66
Development
    cognitive, 55–56
    communication and, 54–55
    Erikson's theory of, 60–67
    growth and, 70–71
    of growth skills, 22
    of insight, 23–24
    psychoanalytic theory of, 56–60
    psychosexual stages of, 58–60
Developmental disabilities, 192, 194
Diagnostic testing, 235
Diet
    culture and, 140, 141
    encouraging, 85
    nutrition and, 218–223
    serving size and, 222–223
    stress and, 184
Dietary guidelines, 221–223
Dignity
    adolescents and, 79
    older patients and, 90

Disabilities
    definition of, 190
    developmental, 192
    mobility, 191
    therapeutic techniques with,
      192–194
    types of, 190–192
Disc, 257*t*
Disciplinary actions, 278
Disclosures, legally required, 123
Disp, 257*t*
Displacing anger, 113
Diversity, 135. *see also* culture
Do not resuscitate (DNR) order, 91
Document composition, 247
Domestic violence, 201–202
Drug addiction, 167–171
DW, 257*t*

E

EDC, 257*t*
Editing, 251
Education, of patients, 209–211
Effective feedback, 17
Ego, 57–58, 59
Ego ideal, 58
Ego integrity *vs.* despair, 65–66
Eight stages, in Erikson, 61–66
Elder abuse, 202, 203
E-mail, 262–264
Emergencies, 231–233
Emotional abuse, 199–200, 203
Emotional characteristics, 13
Emotional self, 6
Empathy
    definition of, 10
    with older patients, 92
    grief and, 178
    importance of, 10
    interpersonal skills and, 23
Empowerment
    of others, 11
    self-esteem and, 10–11
Energy, depression and, 196
Engagement, listening and, 43
Environment
    with adults, 84
    with children, 75
    for patient interviews,
      97–98
Epigenetic principle, 61
Erikson, Erik, 60–67, 69
Et, 257*t*

Exclamation point, 244
Exercise
    active, 225
    anger and, 190
    benefits of, 224
    circulation and, 224–225
    definition of, 224
    encouraging, 85
    importance of, 223
    passive, 225
    physician clearance for,
      225–226
    stress and, 184, 215, 217, 224
    types of, 225
    weight and, 224
Expectations, grief and, 177
Explanations, 83
Ext, 257*t*
Eye contact
    listening and, 43
    verbal communication and, 36
Eye level, with children, 74

F

Face-to-face meetings, 31
Facial expression
    anger and, 187
    nonverbal communication and,
      37–39
Family
    addiction and, 170–171
    in African-American culture,
      145
    in Asian culture, 145
    in Caucasian culture, 144
    in Hawaiian culture, 148–149
    in Hispanic culture, 146
    interactions, 149–150
    in Native American culture,
      147–148
    in Puerto Rican culture, 147
Family history, 102
Fax machine, 265
Federal Child Abuse Prevention
  and Treatment Act, 205
Feedback
    consistency and, 16
    effective, 17
    frequency of, 15
    ineffective, 17
    learning and, 15–16
    message and, 32
    negative, 33

positive, 17, 32–33
  self-concept and, 14–15
  sender and, 15
Feelings, acknowledging, 49
Fever, 107
FGW, 257t
Folk healers, 143
Follow-up, 105
Food, culture and, 141
Food Guide Pyramid, 218, *220*, 222
Formal operational thought, 56
Frequency, of feedback, 15
Freud, Sigmund, 56–60, 69
Friendliness, 23
Fruits, 219
Frustration, 286
FU, 257t

G

G, 257t
Generativity *vs.* stagnation, 65
Genital stage of development, 60
Genuine speech, 12
Geographic location, 159
Geriatric patients. *see* elderly patients
Gm, 257t
Goals, communication, 47
Gossip, 276
Grains, 219
Grammar, 245–247
Grief, 150, 171–179
Grief stages, 171–174
Growth
  communication and, 54–55
  developing skills for, 22
  development and, 70–71
  professional, 297–299
Gt, 257t

H

H, 257t
Hand gestures, 39
Harassment, 199–205
Hawaiian cultural factors, 148–149
Health beliefs, 140–150
Health Insurance Portability and Accountability Act of 1996 (HIPAA), 101, 117–119
Healthy lifestyles, 211–212

Hearing impairments, 107–110, 192, 193
Hierarchy of needs, 19–22
Hispanic cultural factors, 146–147
History
  family, 102
  medical, 101–102, *129–130*
  social, 102
HIV. *see* human immunodeficiency virus (HIV)
Hobbies, 85
Holistic approach, 71
Holistic medicine, 142
Honesty
  with adolescents, 80
  grief and, 178
  interpersonal skills and, 23
Hospice, 236–237
Hr, 257t
HS, 257t
Human immunodeficiency virus (HIV), 161, 179–183

I

ID, 257t
Id, 57, 59
Ideal self, 6
Identification
  with another, 113
  of problem, 114
  of self, 3–4
Identity, *vs.* role confusion, 64–65
IM, 257t
Impairments. *see* disabilities
Implementation, of treatment plan, 115
Incongruent messages, 41–42
Independence, loss of 174–175
Indifference, 112
Indirect statements, 104
Individual, patient as, 177
Industry *vs.* inferiority, 64
Ineffective feedback, 17
Infancy, self-concept in, 4
Influence
  of self-concept, 5–6
  use of, 12
Influencing others, 10–11
Information release, 121–123
Information sharing, communication and, 27–28
Informed consent, 120–121, 181–182

Initiating treatment, 124
Initiative *vs.* guilt, 62–64
Injections, fear of, 76
Insensitivity, cultural, 157
Insight, development of, 23–24
Intention, verbal communication
    and, 36
Interdisciplinary communications,
    273–274
Intermittent reinforcement, 68
Internet, 260–261
Interpersonal skills, development
    of, 23
Interpreters, 155–156
Interviews
    job, 296–297
    patient, 38, 96–106
Intranet, 261–262
Isokinetic exercise, 215
Isolation, 65
Isometric exercise, 215
Isotonic exercise, 215
IV, 257t

J

Judgments, 51, 79–80

K

Kg, 257t
Kinesics, 39–40
Knowledge, health maintenance and,
    208
Kübler-Ross, Elizabeth, 171–172
Kübler-Ross grief stages, 171–174

L

Language barriers, 106–107, 108
Late patients, 233
Latency stage of development, 60
Layman's terms, 105
Lb, 257t
Learning
    about cultures, 136
    feedback and, 15–16
    health maintenance and, 208
Learning theory
    behavioral, 67–68
    cognitive development, 55–56
Lecturing, 51, 112
Legal issues
    abuse and, 203, 205

advance directives, 91, 119–120
confidentiality, 45, 78, 121
with older patients, 91–92
Health Insurance Portability and
    Accountability Act (HIPAA),
    101, 117–119
with HIV/AIDS, 181–182
required disclosures, 123
subpoenas, 123
Letters, written, 247–252, *250*
Lifestyle, healthy, 211–212
Limbs, artificial, 192
Linguistic competence, 137–138
Listening
    active, 45, 46, 48, 100
    attention and, 43
    to children, 75
    engagement and, 43
    eye contact and, 43
    grief and, 177–179
    nonverbal communication
        and, 44
    openness and, 43–44
    overview of, 42–44
Literacy level, 153–155
Living will, 91
LMP, 257t
Loss, 171–179
Love, as need, 20

M

Mailing letters, 251–252
Maladaptations, 61
Malignancies, in Erikson, 61
Manner, verbal communication
    and, 36
Maslow's hierarchy of needs,
    19–22
Material abuse, 201
Material self, 6
Mcg, 257t
Meals on Wheels, 236
Meat, 221
Medical emergencies, 231–233
Medical history, 101–102, *129–130*
Medical records, 254–258, 259–260
Medication, culture and, 140–141
Medication, dosage, 226–227
Medication, educating patients about,
    226–229
Medication, information sheets, 226
Medication, interactions, 228
Medication, name, 226

Medication, route, 227
Medication, side effects, 227–228
Meeting minutes, 253–254
Memoranda, 252–253
Memory loss, 86
Memory repression, 112–113
Meq, 257*t*
Message
    congruent, 41–42
    context and, 33–34
    definition of, 30
    delivery, 82–83
    "I," 79–80, 81
    incongruent, 41–42
    quality of, 30
    receiver, 32
    sender, 32
    style and, 30
    tone and, 30
    "you," 79–80, 81
Milk, 219
Missed appointments, 234
Misunderstandings, 282
Ml, 257*t*
Mobility impairments, 191
Model behavior, 11–12
Mood, 167
Mood swings, 197
Multidimensional approach, to self-
    concept, 16
Muscle tone, 225
Mutuality, 66

N

NaCl, 257*t*
Native American cultural factors,
    147–148
Natural disasters, 174
Needs
    hierarchy of, 19–22
    of patients, 47
Negative energy, 215–216
Negative feedback, 33
Negative stress, 213–214
Neglect, 200
New patient interviews, 96–106
NH, 257*t*
NKA, 257*t*
Noc, 257*t*
Nontherapeutic techniques, 49–51
Nonthreatening environment, 197
Nonverbal communication
    culture and, 153

    definition of, 37
    facial expression and, 37–39
    grief and, 178
    hand gestures and, 39
    kinesics and, 39–40
    listening and, 44
    paralanguage and, 39
    in patient interviews, 99
    personal space and, 40
    posture and, 40
    self-esteem and, 9
    territoriality and, 41
    touch and, 40
Note of Privacy Practices, 119
NPO, 257*t*
Nutrition, 218–223
Nutrition labels, 221–222

O

Objectives, 84
Observation, 45–46
Office managers, 278–280
Office procedures, 230–236
Office space, 98
Oils, in diet, 221
Older patients
    communicating with, 84–92
    dignity and, 90
    effective speaking with, 87–92
    empathy with, 92
    hierarchy of needs and, 21–22
    issues with, 86–87, 91–92
    legal issues with, 91–92
    memory loss in, 86
    myths about, 88–89
    pace of communication and, 89
    reassurance of, 90
    sense of control in, 87–89
Open-ended questions, 38, 48, 104
Openings, broad, 49
Openness
    grief and, 179
    interpersonal skills and, 23
    listening and, 43–44
Operant conditioning, 68–69, 70
Operational thought, 56
Oral stage of development, 58
Organizational structure, 274–275
Others
    connections to, 8–9
    empowerment of, 11
    influencing, 10–11
    uniqueness of, 9–10

P

Pace, older patients and, 89
Paralanguage, 39
Paraphrasing, 38
Parental acceptance, self-esteem and, 7–8
Parentheses, 245
Parents, adolescent privacy and, 80
Participative management, 291–292
Partner, loss of, 175
Passive exercise, 225
Patients. *see also* children; older patients
    abused, 199–205
    advising, 49–50
    brochures for, 267–269
    concern of, 47
    culture and, 150–152
    defensiveness in, 50
    education of, 209–211, 226–229
    helping, 47
    hierarchy of needs and, 21–22
    holistic approach with, 71
    as individuals, 177
    interviewing, 96–106
    late, 233
    needs of, 47
    operant conditioning and, 70
    self-disclosure and, 46
    terminating relationship with, 124–126
    walk-in, 233
Pavlov, Ivan, 67–68
Period (punctuation), 244
Personal differences, 283–284
Personal identity, 3
Personal information, 119
Personal notes, 242
Personal space, nonverbal communication and, 40
Phallic stage of development, 59
Pharmaceutical information sheets, 226
Phone, 31, 264–265, 266
Physical abuse, 199
Physical characteristics, 13
Piaget, Jean, 55–56, 69
Planning, with adults, 83–84
Pleasure principle, 57
Policies and procedures, culture and, 152–153
Positive atmosphere, 16–18
Positive feedback, 17, 32–33

Positive stress, 213
Possessions, loss of, 174
Posture, 40
Poverty, 159–160
Power of attorney, 91
Preoperational thought, 56
Privacy
    adolescents and, 78
    adults and, 84
    note of practices, 119
Problem identification, 114
Problem-solving skills, 114–116
Procedures, office, 230–236
Professional growth, 297–299
Professionalism, 241–242
Projection, 113
Promotion of health maintenance, 208–212
Pronunciation, 264
Proofreading, 251
Protected health information, 119
Psychoanalysis, 56–60
Psychological abuse, 199, 203
Psychological development factors, 55
Psychological self, 6
Psychosexual stages of development, 58–60
Psychosocial crises, 60–61
Public self, 6
Puerto Rican cultural factors, 147
Punctuation, 244–245

Q

Quality
    of message, 30
    of voice, 34
Question mark, 244
Questions
    closed-ended, 104
    interview, 103–104
    open-ended, 38, 48, 104
Quotation marks, 245

R

Rape, 203
Rationalization, 114
Reactions, 14–16
Reality principle, 57
Reassurance, of older patients, 90
Reassuring clichés, 50–51, 111
Receiver, 32
Records, medical, 254–258

Referrals, 235
Reflecting, 100–101
Reflection, 38
Regression, 113
Rehabilitation facilities, 237
Reinforcement, 68
Relapse, addiction, 171
Relationships, 84
Relaxation techniques, 185, 190, 217
Release, of information, 121–123
Reporting requirements, for abuse,
   203
Repression, 112–113
Required disclosures, 123
Respect
   adolescents and, 79
   communication and, 10
   older patients and, 90
   interpersonal skills and, 23
   in workplace, 46
Responses, 14–16
Rest, stress and, 185
Resume, 292–293
Ritual, culture and, 143
Role, 47
Role confusion, 64–65
Role performance, self-concept
   and, 3
Rudeness, 29

S

Safety, as need, 19–20
Sarcasm, 112, 188
Self-acceptance, development of, 7
Self-actualization, as need, 20
Self-awareness, communication
   and, 2
Self-concept
   acceptance and, 7
   in childhood, 4
   as circular, 14–15
   feedback and, 14–15
   identification and, 3–4
   importance of, 6
   in infancy, 4
   influence of, 5–6
   multidimensional approach to,
     16
   origin of, 4–5
   parts of, 2–3, 6–7
   role of, 8–12
   standards and, 4
   strengths and, 12–14

uniqueness and, 9–10
   verbal communication and, 36
   weaknesses and, 12–14
Self-Determination Act, 119–120
Self-disclosure, 46
Self-esteem
   atmosphere and, 16–18
   behavior modeling and, 11–12
   communication and, 9
   competency and, 7
   connections to others and, 8–9
   empowerment and, 10–11
   foundation of, 7–8
   growth of, 8–12
   as need, 20
   nonverbal communication and, 9
   parental acceptance and, 7–8
   self-concept and, 3
   success and, 7
   uniqueness and, 9–10
   verbal communication and, 9
Self-expectations, grief and, 177
Semicolon, 245
Sender, 32
Sensitivity
   over, 29
   verbal communication and, 37
Sensorimotor activities, 56
Sentence structure, 246
Servant-leadership management, 292
Serving sizes, 222–223
Setting, verbal communication and,
   36–37
7 Habits of Highly Effective People
   (Covey), 22
Sexual abuse, 200–201
Sickle-cell anemia, 161
Side effects, 227–228
Significant other, loss of, 175
Signs, 102
Silence, importance of, 38
Skinner, B. F., 67–69
Sleep
   depression and, 196
   grief and, 176–177
   stress and, 185
Social characteristics, 13
Social development factors, 55
Social history, 102
Social self, 6
Social standards, self-concept and, 4
Social values, 14
Society, abuse in, 201–203
Software, 259

Special diets, 223
Speech impairments, 193
Spell check, 244
Spelling, 242–244
Spousal abuse, 202
Stages, of conflict, 285–287
Stages, of grief, 171–174
Stagnation, 65
Statements, indirect, 104
Stereotypes, 156–157
Strengths, 12–14
Stress, 183–185, 212–217
Stress management, 184–185
Stress reduction, 211–212
Structural differences, 284–285
Style
    adapting, 167
    culture and, 155–156
    message and, 30
Subject changing, 50, 112
Sublimation, 114
Subpoenas, 123
Substance abuse, 167–171
Success, self-esteem and, 7
Suicide, 198–199
Summarization, 38
Superego, 58, 59
Supervisory styles, 290–292
Support, 84
Surgery, 236
Survival, as need, 19
Symbols, 256–257
Sympathy, vs. empathy, 10
Symptoms, 102

T
Team, communication with, 272–274
Team, members of, 273
Terminating physician-patient rela-
    tionship, 124–126
Territoriality, 41
Testing, HIV, 181–182
Text messaging, 31
Therapeutic communication skills,
    23–24
Therapy, for addiction, 170–171
T.H.I.N.K., 22
Threats, 188
Tone
    anger and, 187
    children and, 74
    in interviews, 97
    message and, 30

Touch
    with children, 74
    nonverbal communication and,
        40
    in patient interviews, 99
Toys, with children, 74
Traditions, cultural, 134
Transactions, in HIPAA, 117–119
Treatment initiation, 124
Treatment plans, 115
Trust, in interviews, 106
Trust vs. mistrust, in Erikson, 62
TTY, 265–267

U
Undoing, 113
Uniqueness, self-esteem and, 9–10
Unresolved grief, 175–176

V
Values
    cultural, 134
    social, 14
Valuing diversity, 135
Vegetables, 219
Verbal communication
    attitude and, 37
    confidence and, 37
    definition of, 34
    eye contact and, 36
    intention and, 36
    manner and, 36
    self-concept and, 36
    self-esteem and, 9
    sensitivity and, 37
    setting and, 36–37
    voice quality and, 34
Video conferencing, 31
Violence
    criminal, 201
    domestic, 201–202
Visual impairments, 191–192,
    192–193
Visualization, 217
Vocal paralanguage, 39
Voice quality, 34

W
Walk-in patients, 233
Warmth, 23
Water, importance of, 85

Weaknesses, 12–14, 113
Webcasting, 31
Wheelchairs, 193
Work environment, 18
Workplace conflict, 280–285
Workplace dynamics, 274–280
Written communication
    accuracy in, 247
    agendas, 253
    e-mail, 262–264
    grammar and, 245–247
    letters, 247–252, *250*
    medical records, 254–258
    meeting minutes, 253–254
    memoranda, 252–253
    professionalism and, 241–242
    punctuation and, 244–245
    spelling and, 242–244

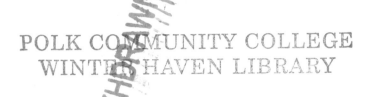